Drink Your Carbs

Drink Your Carbs

eat. drink. sweat. REPEAT

STEVEN DEUTSCH and ANDREA SEEBAUM

DYC LLC
San Francisco, CA

DYC LLC
584 Castro Street #824
San Francisco, CA 94114
info@drinkyourcarbs.com

ISBN: 978-0-9904496-0-7 (hardcover)
ISBN: 978-0-9904496-1-4 (paperback)
ISBN: 978-0-9904496-2-1 (ePub e-book)
ISBN: 978-0-9904496-3-8 (Kindle e-book)

Cover Design by Misa Erder.
Interior Design by Jennifer Omner.
Illustrations by Nicole Delmage, Mike Jenson and Boyd Richard.
The photograph of Steven and Andrea in Crete was taken by Tricia Tilley.

[Insert Mandatory Warning Here]—Seriously? We have to warn people to check with their doctor before making changes to their eating, drinking and exercise plans? If they can't figure that out on their own we should probably go back through the book and remove all the big words.

Contents

Introduction What Is Drink Your Carbs? 1

One How Diets Work 11

Two Why Are Americans Fat? 27

Three The Drink Your Carbs Food Pyramid 37

Four Three Simple Steps to Get Started Now 39

Five The Basic Drink Your Carbs Diet 45

Six The Basic Drink Your Carbs Food List 51

Seven Austerity Mode 75

Eight The Austerity Mode Food List 81

Nine Nightmare Mode 85

Ten How to Cheat on Your Diet 89

Eleven Grading Your Performance 95

Twelve Maintenance 97

Thirteen What about Gluten and Dairy? 101

Fourteen Alcohol and Other Beverages 107

Fifteen How Much Can I Drink? 117

Sixteen Artificial and Alternative Sweeteners 125

Seventeen Sports Drinks 129

Eighteen Don't Drive Drunk 133

Nineteen Exercise: A Necessary Evil 135

Twenty Basic Exercise 139

Twenty One Advanced Exercise 147

Twenty Two Insane Exercise 161

Twenty Three Incorporating Exercise into Your Life 177

Twenty Four Travel 185

Twenty Five Travel Case Study: Las Vegas, Nevada 187

Twenty Six Travel Case Study: New York, New York 203

Twenty Seven Travel Case Study: Antarctica 211

Twenty Eight Travel Case Study: Middle East 223

Twenty Nine Travel Case Study: Crete, Greece 231

Thirty Case Study 243

Thirty One A History of Drinker's Diets 247

Thirty Two Recipes 257
Three Awesome Salad Dressings 259
Raw Kale Salad 266
The Burger Salad 270
Chicken alla Milanese 278
Easy Green Sauce 283
Perfect Kale 289
Easy Black Beans 292
Drink Your Carbs Brownies 295

Thirty Three Cocktails 299
The Drink Your Carbs Margarita 302
The Amaro Cocktail 303
Bartender's Guide to Mixing Unimaginative Drinks 305
A Love Letter to Perfect Cocktail Ice 309

Blooper Reel 313

Acknowledgments 319

Notes 323

About the Authors 335

Introduction

What Is Drink Your Carbs?

The short answer: Drink Your Carbs is a how-to guide for losing weight without giving up alcohol.

The long answer is more complex.

We never intended to write a diet book. Drink Your Carbs began as a joke. In many ways, it is still a joke. It just happens to be a joke diet that works.

Drink Your Carbs began back in 2008 with a friendly competition between co-author Steven and his childhood friend Chris. They were both approaching 40 and, like most of their peers, had begun to put on weight. Chris was the first to declare he wanted to reverse the trend. More specifically, Chris wanted six-pack abs. He wanted to be ripped and he wanted it to happen before his 39th birthday. That way he could cruise into 40 in the best shape of his life.

Chris was in no way obese. He had somewhere between 15 and 20 pounds to lose. The magic of a six pack is that you have no idea at what weight it will suddenly appear, or if it will appear at all. Visible abdominal muscles are very much genetic. The only way to find out if it's in your DNA is to slim down.

Chris had four months to meet his goal. The timeline was aggressive. It would not be easy, but Chris knew that if he stayed disciplined, four months would be more than enough time to lose the spare tire that he had spent most of a decade building.

When Chris called Steven to share his plan, the conversation went something like this:

> **Chris**: I'm doing it. Washboard abs in four months. I'm upping the intensity of my workouts. I'll do two-a-days, cardio in the morning, weights in the afternoon. I'm also cutting all the carbs out of my diet.
>
> **Steven**: I hear your challenge and I accept. I'll do the same. We'll meet somewhere in December, run a half marathon and at the finish shirts come off.
>
> **Chris**: I'm also going to stop drinking.
>
> **Steven**: What!? Why would you do that?
>
> **Chris**: You have to cut the carbs if you want to lose weight.
>
> **Steven**: I'm still in. But just to piss you off, I'm going to keep drinking.
>
> **Chris**: I don't think that's going to work.
>
> **Steven**: You'll see. I'll lose just as much weight as you do.

Everyone expected Chris would win.

Steven and Chris ran the half marathon in Las Vegas. They chose Vegas because it was cheap to get to and hosts one of the few races scheduled at the end of the year. Chris won the footrace by a huge margin. By the time Steven wheezed his way across the finish, Chris had been waiting for nearly an hour in the sponsored beer tent. It was not yet 8 a.m. The combination of not drinking for four months and low electrolytes from the race meant that Chris was in rare form. He was happy. He was smiling. He was in love with the whole world. As he cheered Steven across the finish line, strangers edged away.

After the race, shirts came off. Unfortunately, no one thought to take "before" photos. The "after" shots offer no perspective on how far they came, but they do show a couple of guys looking pretty good for their age. They both lost similar amounts of weight in spite of their differing strategies. They both lost a few belt notches. In both cases, the results were outwardly apparent. Friends and family were stunned by their transformations.

Chris unanimously won the flex-off, although several of the judges contend that Chris won largely because he knew how to flex. Chris moved smoothly from pose to pose, showing off his new physique. Steven had spent hours practicing in front of a mirror yet when it came time for competition he pretty much threw his hands up over his head like he was protecting himself from falling objects.

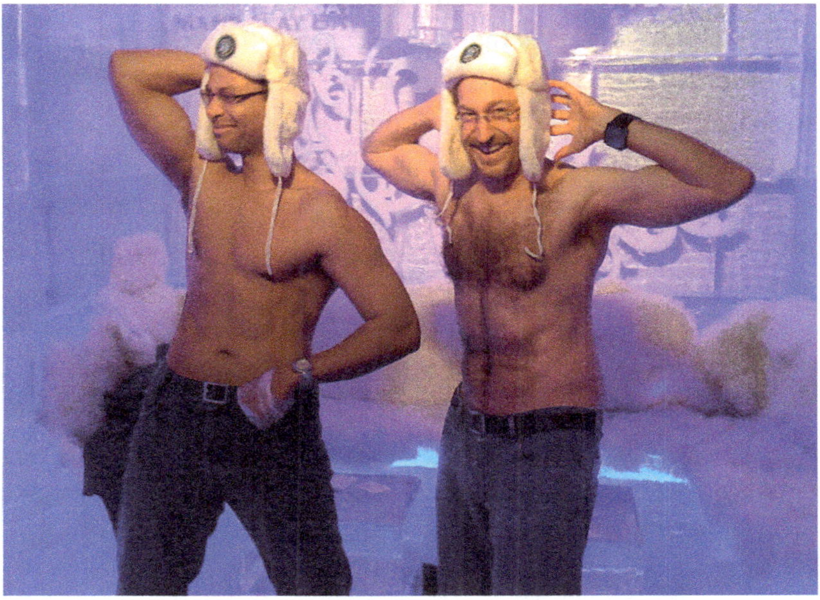

Steven is the hairy one in the awkward pose.

Andrea, who is both co-author of this book and married to Steven, also followed the low-carb, drinking diet over those same four months. Although Andrea didn't compete in the posedown, she also lost weight. In spite of the fact that Andrea had far less to lose, she emerged from the competition over five pounds lighter.

The diet Steven and Andrea followed evolved into Drink Your Carbs.

At its core, it's a diet built on calorie restriction. We strongly believe that all successful diets are methods of calorie restriction. This is because gaining and losing weight comes down to a simple equation: calories in versus calories out. If you burn more calories than you consume, you lose weight. If you consume more calories than you burn, you gain weight.

This is true regardless of whether you live on unsalted vegetables or pure bacon fat. This is true whether you eat like a Neanderthal or eat only shrink-wrapped foods manufactured in the industrial food labs that line the Jersey Turnpike. Vegetables or meat. Raw or cooked. Organic or irradiated. It's even true if most of your calories come from high-fructose corn syrup; if this sounds impossible, suspend your disbelief until you've read the case study on nutritionist Mark Haub in Chapter One. Some diets are unquestionably healthier than others, but the simple calories-in/calories-out arithmetic determines weight gain or loss.

What about the Calories in Alcohol?

There is no shortage of experts who delight in pointing out that half a bottle of wine with dinner adds roughly 300 to 325 calories to your day; a couple of pints of microbrew can add even more. The calories in alcohol, they argue, are too high and therefore incompatible with any form of dieting.

These prohibitionists are making a simple assumption: that the calories in alcohol are purely additive. In other words, they assume that people will make no other changes to their diet beyond adding a few drinks. Under this theory, the calories in alcohol are like the rainbow sprinkles on a banana split; they are excessive and unnecessary.

The no-alcohol crowd holds similar beliefs regarding exercise. They assume that few people will make any effort to burn off those extra calories. Recent statistics support their assumption. According to a study by a team of researchers at Penn State University, the average American between the ages of 18 and 64 gets only 17 minutes of exercise per day.[1] Shockingly, this includes as exercise walking across a parking lot from your car into an ice-cream parlor.

Drink Your Carbs is based on very different assumptions.

We are not in denial about the calories in alcoholic drinks. We trust the validity of the exercise figures from Penn State. We fully acknowledge the hideous state of the American nutrition and fitness landscape. The difference is that we refuse to hang our heads in defeat and declare alcohol forever unworkable. Instead, we celebrate the current state of American health because it makes Drink Your Carbs easily doable for nearly everyone.

The whole point of Drink Your Carbs is that if you want lose weight while continuing to drink, the calories you consume in alcohol must be burned and/or offset. We are also adamant that these calories be eliminated without sacrificing the quantity of food eaten or daily nutrition. The dreadful state of the American diet makes this as easy as pie.

Fact: According to the American Heart Association the average American eats 22 teaspoons of sugar per day. This represents 355 utterly empty calories.[2] There is no denying that Americans mainline sugar with the same unbridled lust that Amy Winehouse brought to a brand new dime bag.

> Those of us who don't drink sodas or eat candy bars should not get cocky. Most of us still consume way too many high-calorie, low-nutrition foods.

Over the past 50 years, heavily processed foods have come to dominate the American diet. It's often said that a true American cuisine is hard to define; we think that the single most defining attribute is too many empty calories. The second most defining characteristic is probably the color beige.

> **Fact:** The American diet, with all its related health problems, is one of the nation's most successful exports. If you're a fan of conspiracy theories, a strong argument can be made that America is in the process of taking over the world, one case of Type-2 Diabetes at a time.

Drink Your Carbs is designed to help you identify these empty calories and eliminate them. We will show you that by making simple changes to your existing diet and exercise routine there is room for alcohol in your weight-loss plan.

There is no magic. There are no pills to take nor proprietary shakes to blend. There is no need to embarrass yourself at weekly weigh-ins or purchase Drink Your Carbs-branded frozen dinners. The Drink Your Carbs concept is simple: the calories in alcohol can be offset through a combination of exercise and exchanging high-calorie, low-nutrition foods such as added sugars and simple carbohydrates for quality meats, fresh fruit and vegetables.

Make no mistake: Drink Your Carbs is a low-carbohydrate diet in that it contains far fewer and far healthier carbs than you'll find in the typical American's diet. But Drink Your Carbs is about more than just reducing carbs; it is heavily informed by calories in versus calories out. This makes Drink Your Carbs far from a typical low-carb diet.

Nowhere in all of our discussions of food will you find permission to live on bacon, mayonnaise and pastrami sandwiched between two pieces of brie. Nor will we recommend tossing aside nonfat milk in favor of heavy cream in your coffee. Heavy cream may be low in carbs, but ounce for ounce it packs nine times more calories. Low-carb breads, pretzels, pancake mixes, crumb cakes and cookies may be acceptable on traditional low-carb diets, but not on Drink Your Carbs. We don't care if these products have been engineered to be low in carbohydrates. There are some things you just don't eat, especially food that delivers little nutritional benefit while often containing more calories than two pints of Guinness.

Nor will you be allowed to gulp down unlimited piña coladas in celebration of your new diet. A piña colada is the caloric equivalent of drinking a shot of rum with a banana split on the side. If you want to lose weight while continuing to drink, sacrifices will have to be made. Some drinks, such as piña coladas, have to be eliminated altogether. When choosing between a 97-calorie shot of tequila and a 400-calorie, day-glo margarita, you will learn to pick the shot. This is the price that must be paid.

> **Fact:** You can still enjoy cocktails in a mixer-free world. We not only provide drink recipes, we have included a condensed bartender's guide to mixing Drink Your Carbs-compliant cocktails.

To make the task simpler we created the Drink Your Carbs Food List, a comprehensive list of what should be eaten, limited or altogether avoided. There is no need to keep a food journal or download a carb counter to your phone. Eat and drink according to the rules of the Food List and your caloric intake will drop even though you will likely be eating more. There are plenty of options to keep your diet both diverse and interesting. Don't even think about portions. All we ask is that you stick to the Food List and stop eating when you feel full.

> **Fact:** Finishing your plate does nothing to help starving children in Africa. Stop eating when you feel full and make a donation to the aid organization of your choice.

Furthermore, our exercise recommendations will send your calorie burn skyrocketing. Exercise will be covered in detail. For now, we will simply caution that "exercise" does not include the "Executive Workout" where your hang out in the gym talking to friends, do a couple of reps on a bench press machine and head to the steam room. Exercise requires a serious routine that elevates your heart rate for at least 20 minutes and burns significant calories. This is the absolute minimum.

If you follow our food and exercise program, you will have no problem burning through and/or offsetting the calories in wine, beer or even the hard stuff.

We believe Drink Your Carbs is the most easy-to-follow diet you will ever find. Drink Your Carbs is not a temporary solution. You will not live in constant state of denial. You will not be hungry. You'll get plenty of food and have plenty of energy. Exercising and eating well will leave you feeling great. Above all else, you will not have to give up happy hour. Drink Your Carbs allows you to continue to enjoy a social life while cutting calories and losing weight.

Drink Your Carbs began as a joke and turned out to be a surprisingly effective diet. We never set out to create it. It was an accidental discovery. All of the changes and refinements we have made were the direct result of tweaking the diet for our own needs. We were, and still are, our own lab rats.

It has been six years since the shirtless flex-off in Las Vegas and Steven has yet to regain any of the weight he lost. Sure, the hair on top of his head has migrated to his back and shoulders, but he still wears the same sized pants. This is due entirely to Drink Your Carbs.

> **Fact:** Drink Your Carbs is only responsible for Steven's pants size. The body hair is the fault of his Eastern European ancestry.

A Final Word of Warning: As Americans, we feel it necessary to add warning labels to everything. These warnings are as much a part of our legal system as powdered wigs are to the British or extra-judicial killings are to those little countries that used to be part of the Soviet Union. We have actually seen a warning label on a frozen dinner reading, "Caution: After Cooking, Contents May Be Hot."

In this grand American tradition, we offer our warning: talk to your doctor before starting any diet or exercise program. We recommend a very lean diet and some pretty intense workouts. Even if you're in optimal health, significantly altering your eating, drinking and exercising habits can have unpredictable effects. In some cases, it can even be outright dangerous. Before undertaking any of our recommendations, confirm with your doctor that you're not doing something stupid.

Drink Your Carbs has not been tested on animals. We did not even test it on a single gerbil. If we had tested it on a gerbil, for all we know the gerbil would have died. Almost certainly no one would have cleaned its cage.

Drink Your Carbs is designed for people of legal drinking age.

And finally, if you have a drinking problem, by all means get help and find a diet that prohibits drinking. Drink Your Carbs contains great advice for drinkers who want to lose weight. But this is absolutely the worst advice possible for people who can't control their drinking and/or have taken the step of giving up alcohol altogether. Alcoholics should stay away from Drink Your Carbs for the same reasons that vegans should avoid Atkins. Not every diet is appropriate for every dieter.

One

How Diets Work

There are as many opinions about dieting as there are books, articles and websites on the subject. Not only are there thousands of recommendations, they are contradictory and mutually exclusive. Every so-called diet expert would have you believe that his or hers is the only approach that works and that every other method or philosophy is downright dangerous.

Advocates for low-fat diets insist that high protein, low-carb diets don't work, cause cancer and are responsible for everything from heart disease to the national debt. The equally credentialed authors of low-carb diets blame the much higher-carb, low-fat diets for the exact same list. Even authors within the same dieting category take shots at one another. Reading competing diet books is like taking a high school class in comparative religion. These authors take the same essentialist position as most faiths. They control the keys to heaven. Everyone else is knowingly trying to lead you astray.

We'll let the experts speak for themselves.

Robert Atkins—The Atkins Diet versus All

By far the best-known advocate for a low-carb diet was Dr. Robert Atkins. In his book, *New Diet Revolution* Dr. Atkins placed the blame for American obesity squarely on the shoulders of promoters for low-fat diets. "The influential but, alas, ineffective school of low-fat dieting . . . has been the dominant trend in dieting for the past decade, but its dominance hasn't, by and large, done a thing to take the pounds off . . . [L]ow-fat dieting . . . is a major national embarrassment."[1]

Dean Ornish—The Dean Ornish Diet versus Atkins

In an article for *The Huffington Post*, Dr. Dean Ornish, who is arguably the reigning king of the low-fat approach, wrote, "I've been saying [this] all along: an Atkins diet is not healthful and may shorten your lifespan."[2]

Nathan Pritkin—The Permanent Weight-Loss Manual versus Atkins

In his *Pritikin Permanent Weight-Loss Manual*, low-fat guru Nathan Pritikin made no effort to hide his disdain for Atkins and other low-carb diets. "These diets simply are not safe," Pritikin wrote. He went on to accuse Atkins of knowingly and intentionally damaging the health of his followers.[3]

Arthur Agatson—The South Beach Diet versus Pritikin and Ornish

In his book, *The South Beach Diet*, Dr. Arthur Agatston advocates a low-carb approach. In his introduction, he notes that early in his career he enthusiastically championed "Pritikin and the [other] heart-healthy low-fat regimens, including the Ornish plan . . . " Dr. Agatston abandoned the low-fat approach after, "[e]ach of them, for different reasons, failed miserably. Either the diets were too difficult to stick with, or the promise of improved blood chemistry and cardiac heath remained just that—a promise."[4]

It is no wonder that dieters have trouble sorting through the data.

We strongly believe that all diets works work on the same principle: calories in versus calories out. We do not believe that certain categories of foods are to blame for obesity. The law of conservation of mass causes obesity. Matter cannot be created nor destroyed. If you eat more than your body can convert to energy, the remainder is stored. This would be awesome news if you could burn all of that stored energy at once in a giant burst of speed. Unfortunately, that's not how it works. Usain Bolt is at no risk of having his world record time in the 100-meter dash broken by someone who is morbidly obese.

What Exactly Is a Calorie?

The less-than-helpful, highly technical answer: one calorie is the amount of heat required to raise one gram of water one degree Celsius. Calories are not specific to food. Any combustible material contains measurable calories. At the high end, a gallon of gasoline contains over 31 million calories. A standard ballpoint pen contains far fewer. This is an educated guess. We have been unable to find someone willing to throw his or her pen into a bomb calorimeter in order to accurately calculate this number.

Which brings us to the best-named piece of scientific equipment ever: the bomb calorimeter.

This is the machine into which any object from a Twinkie to a ballpoint pen can be placed and burned in order to measure its calories. We're shocked that no one has tried to change the name. These days, simple Googling the words "bomb calorimeter" is probably enough to trigger some automated government spy system to add your name to the TSA No-Fly List.

With a name like bomb calorimeter, it has to look cool. And believe us, they look as cool as they sound. Picture an old-fashioned whiskey still attached to a vintage tube amplifier. Some even display the calories in the same red, LCD letters as 1970s alarm clocks. There are, of course, modern companies manufacturing bomb calorimeters encased in plastic that look like oversized laser printers; we think the labs that buy these have no sense of style.

Food, or any other organic material, is placed into a sealed glass cylinder and lowered into a tank of water in the center of the bomb calorimeter. The contents of the cylinder are then ignited using an electrical current. This process gives off heat that is absorbed by the water surrounding the cylinder. The amount of heat varies based on what was burned in the cylinder. The calories are determined by the rise in the water temperature. The higher the number of calories in the material being burned, the warmer the water gets. The remnants of whatever was in the cylinder typically look like the aftermath of the worst Fourth of July barbeque ever. Hotdogs are distinguishable from hamburgers only by shape. If you try to go by taste, neither is distinguishable from the pen.

These days, bomb calorimeters are rarely used for measuring the calories in food. The current standard food industry methodology involves plugging the ingredients and quantities into a database of food ingredients. The database not only spits out the calories, but all of the information required for the nutritional label. We have no idea how the accuracy of this new system compares to the old one.

These databases are proprietary and owned by the food manufacturers and trade organizations. Not only does this sound like a massive conflict of interest, it also means that we cannot directly evaluate the data. The most we can say is that having a database estimate your calories sounds a little having your Body Mass Index measured by the weight guesser at the circus. Those guys can be eerily accurate, but the process is far from a reliable replacement for being measured in a doctor's office.

> **Fact:** To confuse matters further, the calories listed on food packages are not calories, but kilocalories. A kilocalorie is 1,000 calories. Anything edible is measured in kilocalories; everything else is measured in regular calories. This is not difficult math to do, but you'll have to take it into account if you want to compare the calories in a ballpoint pen to those in a Hostess Cherry Pie.

So, a calorie is a measurement of the heat given off by food as it's burned to a tiny lump of carbon. But is a calorie a calorie? Does this mean that 100 calories in carrots is wholly equivalent to 100 calories in high-fructose corn syrup? For the past 30 years, the answer would've been an unqualified yes. Obviously, the carrots are healthier and contain more nutritional value. But when it came to calculating calories consumed, both types of calories were considered to have an equal impact on a dieter's waistline.

Are All Calories Equal?

There's an emerging body of research that purports to show that some calories are worse than others in terms of causing obesity. A good example is a recent study conducted at Princeton University comparing rats fed high-fructose corn syrup to rats fed sucrose from sugar cane and sugar beets. Not surprisingly, both groups of sugar-junkie rats gained weight. However, in spite of the fact that they all consumed the same number of calories, the rats fed high-fructose corn syrup gained more weight. This was a small study that lasted only a few months. The findings have yet to be verified by other studies. But if the results hold, this insight has the potential to change the way calories are measured.[5]

We wouldn't be surprised to learn that high-fructose corn syrup packs a greater punch than other sugars when it comes to weight gain in laboratory rats or even people. The human body is not a bomb calorimeter. We don't actually burn food for fuel. Instead, nutrients are broken down through dozens of different metabolic pathways. It makes perfect sense that it might take more energy to break down 100 calories in carrots than 100 calories in high-fructose corn syrup. Ideally, the calorie count we use for food would take this into account.

Net calories—raw calories minus the amount of energy it takes for the average person to break a food down—would be a far more useful measure of the value of what we are actually consuming and its impact on the body. Assuming the Princeton study is duplicated, the calories listed for high-fructose corn syrup should probably rise, while the calories in other sugars might drop slightly. This would allow consumers to make more accurate comparisons between foods. While we realize that most people ignore calories altogether, we always come down on the side of providing more accurate information.

The studies we've seen so far have only compared the effects of high-fructose corn syrup with sucrose. We have yet to see anyone compare high-fructose corn syrup with carrots. In fact, every major food would have to be evaluated before nutritional labels could carry net calories. We're a long way from this happening. For now, we have to rely on old-fashioned calories—technically kilocalories—as determined by a proprietary database that one must assume mirrors the results of actually detonating foods in a bomb calorimeter.

Fact: All of the Princeton rats that were fed sugar gained weight. If you're the kind of person who changes his or her behavior based on the latest research study, keep in mind that the only rats that did not gain weight were in the control group. If you want to emulate their behavior you should drink only water and eat only rat chow.

Also worth mentioning, if you attend Princeton and you're looking for a name for your a cappella group, you could do far worse than The Princeton Rats.

Even if the calories on packaged foods labels are changed to reflect net calories, we do not believe that the difference will be large enough to form a new dieting philosophy. Substituting Coke made with high-fructose corn syrup for the Mexican variety containing cane sugar will never be a viable weight-loss strategy. The difference between the two sugars is simply not large enough. In the end, successful dieting will continue to come down to the quantity of calories consumed, not the type.

For anyone who still believes that the type of calories is more important than the quantity we offer the case study of Mark Haub, a man who spent two months on the least healthy diet imaginable.

Case Study, the Junk Food Diet: Mark Haub teaches nutrition at Kansas State University. In 2010, Haub undertook a personal experiment where for two months, two-thirds of his calories came in the form of junk food. And no one can accuse Haub of gaming the system by picking healthier junk food options. He ate foods we wouldn't throw into our compost bin. The vast majority of his calories came from Cheetos, Little Debbie Devil Cremes, Sno-Balls, Oreos, Ding Dongs and the like.

The final third of Haub's calories came in the form of canned vegetables (less than a can per day), a protein shake and a multi-vitamin. By all measurements, Haub's diet made Morgan Spurlock's *Supersize Me* McDonalds regime look downright balanced.

Before Haub began his experiment, he was not a small guy. By the Body Mass Index standard that he taught to his students, he was obese.

What makes Haub's diet unique is that he limited himself to 1,800 calories per day. He estimates that, before he began the junk food diet, he was consuming 2,600 calories per day. In other words, the junk food diet was a dramatic reduction in daily calories even though it was an increase in foods that most of us would rank somewhere between unhealthy and outright harmful. If the kind and quality of calories were more important than the number of calories consumed, Haub should have continued putting on weight.

We were not surprised to learn that Haub lost 27 pounds over the course of the two months. Consuming 800 fewer calories per day was a huge reduction. His calorie burn stayed roughly the same. Assuming weight loss really is based on the equation calories in versus calories out, the results were predictable. He should have lost weight, and he did. There is nothing special or magic about his diet. Any diet that restricted his calories to the same level would have yielded a similar result.

Just because Haub lost weight doesn't make the junk food diet a good idea. We were planning a long tirade about how packaged foods from gas stations and vending machines are the opposite of healthy eating. But that rant is unnecessary because of Haub's self-imposed prohibition. The junk food diet included no alcohol. He didn't drink a single glass of wine or beer during the course of his experiment. So instead of an impassioned plea about the importance of consuming real foods with nutritional density, we'll simply write off the junk food diet as incompatible with the Drink Your Carbs lifestyle.[6]

All successful diets follow the same model. Atkins, Ornish, South Beach, Weight Watchers, Deal-a-Meal, Jenny Craig and even Slim Fast are all strategies to reduce overall caloric intake. In the case of Jenny Craig and Slim Fast, this is easy to see. Both diets limit your calories by selling you most of the food you consume. They prepare the food. They define the portions. The end result is a dramatic reduction in calories.

Dr. Dean Ornish and other advocates of low-fat diets readily admit that their approach dramatically decreases the number of calories eaten. The low-fat approach not only limits fatty meats, which are higher calorie than lean meats, but also bans most processed foods, fried foods and added sugars. This alone is enough to reduce a typical American's calories to where he or she will begin losing weight.

Fact: Dr. Ornish has never eaten even a single french fry. If he had, we would have seen the video on YouTube.

Weight Watchers takes a different approach to calorie restriction. Instead of prohibiting certain foods, the program discourages high-calorie foods by converting all meals and snacks to points and then saddling higher-calorie foods with a punitive point cost. Since you get a limited number of food points per day, if you eat a Twinkie you might find yourself lacking enough points for dinner.

Atkins and other low-carb diets also reduce calories, but the method by which they do so is far less obvious. The key to their approach is that the highest-calorie foods most of us consume are simple carbohydrates including all forms of sugar, bread, pasta, rice and potatoes. Adherents to Atkins, South Beach and the other low-carb diets eat close to none of these foods.

While it is true that some low-carb diets allow dieters to eat unlimited quantities of bacon and full-fat sour cream, few people are capable of eating those foods in quantities high enough to come close to their pre-diet caloric intake. Consider this: in order to match the calories in a McDonalds' lunch consisting of a Big Mac, large fries and a Coke you would have to choke down a full pound of New York steak topped with more than a cup of sour cream. If you prefer, for the same calories as in the McDonalds' Extra Value Meal, you could instead gorge yourself on an entire package of bacon and still have over 600 calories left for lunch.

> **Fact:** Unless you are champion speed eater Joey Chestnut—who recently showed himself capable of consuming 66 hotdogs in 12 minutes—it is nearly impossible to eat as many calories in fatty foods as it is in simple sugars and carbohydrates.

Without carbohydrates to make it palatable, there is a limit to the fat most people can consume. While Atkins allows unlimited butter, actual butter consumption ends up limited by the fact that there is no bread to smear it on. Atkins allows unlimited fatty meats but permits no noodles, potatoes, buns or rice to soak up the grease. If you insist on eating everything on your plate, you will have to go after the pan drippings with a spoon. Consider also that Atkins forbids dessert, since the diet eliminates nearly all sugar. A large piece of cake or a crème brûlée can clock in at 500 calories; adherents to the Atkins diet consume none of these. Atkins may allow virtually unlimited fat, but in exchange it eliminates all of the other common sources of high-density calories.

It is also worth mentioning that the goal of most low-carb diets is to force your body into a state called ketosis. By dropping dietary carbohydrates to near zero, the body is forced to burn fat for energy. Recent evidence indicates that entering a state of ketosis speeds up a dieter's metabolism and results in faster weight loss.[7] Another study, however, found no significant difference in weight loss after two years on either a low-carb or low-fat diet.[8] In other words, any advantage from ketosis appears to vanish over a relatively short timeline. In the end, dieting success still requires a reduction in calories.

Fact: We actively encourage dieters to consume enough healthy fruit and vegetable carbs to stay out of ketosis. This puts us at odds with traditional low-carb dieting.

In the 1992 edition of *Dr. Atkins' New Diet Revolution*, Dr. Atkins described ketosis as "one of life's charmed gifts. It's as delightful as sex and sunshine, and it has fewer drawbacks than either of them."[9]

We have no idea what else Dr. Atkins was up to while having sex or hanging out in light of day, but the known side effects of ketosis include nausea, fatigue,

> headaches, bad breath, oily stool and, according to some researchers, permanent kidney damage. Setting aside the possibility of kidney damage because there is conflicting research on the subject, it is worth pointing out that a dieter's initial reaction to entering a ketogenic state can be so severe that it is referred to in the Atkins' community as the "Induction Flu."
>
> To clarify our position and head off some of the hate mail from the low-carb mafia: the reason we do not encourage ketosis has nothing to do with health and everything to do with the side effects. Why experience discomfort when it is entirely unnecessary for achieving one's long-term weight loss goals?

Even diet pills rely on the same basic principle of calories in versus out.

There are two types of diet pills on the market, even though the pharmaceutical industry tries to divide them into more categories. The first type increases your calorie burn (calories out). These pills are typically marketed under names like "fat burners" and "metabolism boosters." Don't fool yourself. All of these labels are just fancy names for speed.

The second category of pills—the category we refer to as Shit Yourself Thin—reduces calories by preventing your body from absorbing the food you eat. These are the latest trend in weight loss drugs. They work by stopping your body from processing calories. Food passes through you undigested. On paper, not digesting food has a similar effect to not eating it: your caloric intake is reduced.

Unfortunately, no pill has yet defeated thermodynamics, so all of that bulk ends up going right through you. Even the companies that sell these pills admit that, for some people, this process can be awkward. Not surprisingly, the warning labels on these supplements read like the plot of a low-budget horror film.

> **Case Study in Shit Yourself Thin Diets:** We have a friend named Chris M. who decided to lose weight using the fat-blocking drug Orlistat. It works by blocking fat absorption. The fat you consume is pushed undigested through your body. Apparently, in some people, that undigested fat is expelled without notice at the most inopportune times. The most shocking thing is that with all of the marketing money pharmaceutical companies have at their disposal they have been unable to purchase a better name for this side effect than "anal leakage."
>
> Chris M. was so afraid of "anal leakage" that he pretty much stopped eating processed foods. Chris M. eliminated all fried food, as well as most of the other saturated fats in his diet. He went from living off fast food to eating a balanced diet of lean meats and fresh vegetables. Before Chris M. decided to shit himself thin, we cannot recall him ordering a salad. Suddenly salads were the cornerstone of his diet. This incredible transformation can be credited to the fact that Chris M. refused to wear an adult diaper.
>
> Chris M. lost a ton of weight and as a result believes that the Orlistat worked. Considering the radical changes to his diet, we are absolutely certain that a placebo would've been just as effective.

All of these approaches can be successful for weight loss. Again, the reason any diet works is calories in versus calories out (or calories in and out very quickly). Regardless of the philosophy behind the diet, each approach, if followed rigorously, will reduce your caloric intake. Drink Your Carbs works on the same principle. We require exercise to increase your calorie burn. Our Food List is designed to reduce the number of calories you consume.

There is simply no other way to successfully diet. Anyone who tells you otherwise is selling you the dietary equivalent of perpetual motion; their system violates the basic laws of physics and, more importantly, won't work.

This is not to say that all diets are equally effective. Without a doubt some diets work faster than others.

We readily admit that meeting your weight-loss goals on Drink Your Carbs can be slower than on other diets. While other diets either heavily restrict or eliminate alcohol, we embrace it. Those extra calories reduce the calorie deficit generated by Drink Your Carbs. The result is slower weight loss than from diets designed to produce greater calorie deficits.

> **Fact:** Drink Your Carbs is absolutely the wrong choice if you need a diet to help you fit into a bridesmaid dress purchased two sizes too small for a wedding less than a month away. We don't know which diet is the fastest, but it is probably some combination of severe calorie restriction and a Shit Yourself Thin supplement that has to be mail ordered from Canada and packaged in coffee grinds because it has been banned by the FDA.

Slow and steady weight loss is a good thing. Diets designed for rapid weight loss tend to work well for a short period of time. The problem is that no one seems able to stick to them. The Shit Yourself Thin shakes and supplements have too many negative side effects. Severe caloric restriction is impossible to adhere to for any extended period of time. People tend to lose a lot of weight quickly, sometimes as much as a pound a day, and then regain that weight and more. This yo-yo effect, more than anything, explains why at any given time 45 million Americans are on some kind of diet even as the ranks of the obese continue to swell.[10]

> **Fact:** If you choose a diet that makes you feel weak, sick or otherwise contains restrictions and lifestyle changes that you are not able to follow over the long term, you will almost certainly fall off that diet and your weight will almost certainly rebound.

Drink Your Carbs is designed to avoid this trap. In our experience, the knowledge that you will spend the evening relaxing with a drink encourages healthy food choices throughout the day. Allowing yourself to drink makes healthy eating feel less like a burden. Dieters tend to adhere more strictly to Drink Your Carbs than previous diets. It's far easier to skip the pasta and order a salad for lunch when you're looking forward to wine with dinner or an evening out at a bar with friends.

> **Fact:** Happy hour is Drink Your Carbs approved even though the happy hour menu typically is not.

Two

Why Are Americans Fat?

According to the Centers for Disease Control, over one-third of American adults are obese.[1] This begs the simple question: why? There are hundreds of competing theories. Every diet guru points to a different cause. Atkins blames carbs. Dean Ornish blames Atkins. Even our elected officials have gotten involved in the finger pointing. New York City has placed the blame squarely on sodas served in cups larger than 16-ounces. The City of San Francisco has chosen instead to vilify Happy Meal toys.

We have our own theory. We blame the dramatic increase in American obesity on the *USDA Food Pyramid*. We realize that on the surface this sounds a little like blaming Doonesbury for the divisive state of American politics. Nonetheless, we argue that a cartoon pyramid deserves the lion's share of the responsibility for derailing the American diet.

We have vivid memories of growing up in the late 1970s under the dietary autocracy of the *USDA Food Pyramid*. Not the revised *MyPyramid*, which looks like an advertisement for My Little Pony.[2] We're talking about the original Food Pyramid, the one modeled on a combination of the Great Pyramids of Giza and, ever popular at the time, black light posters.

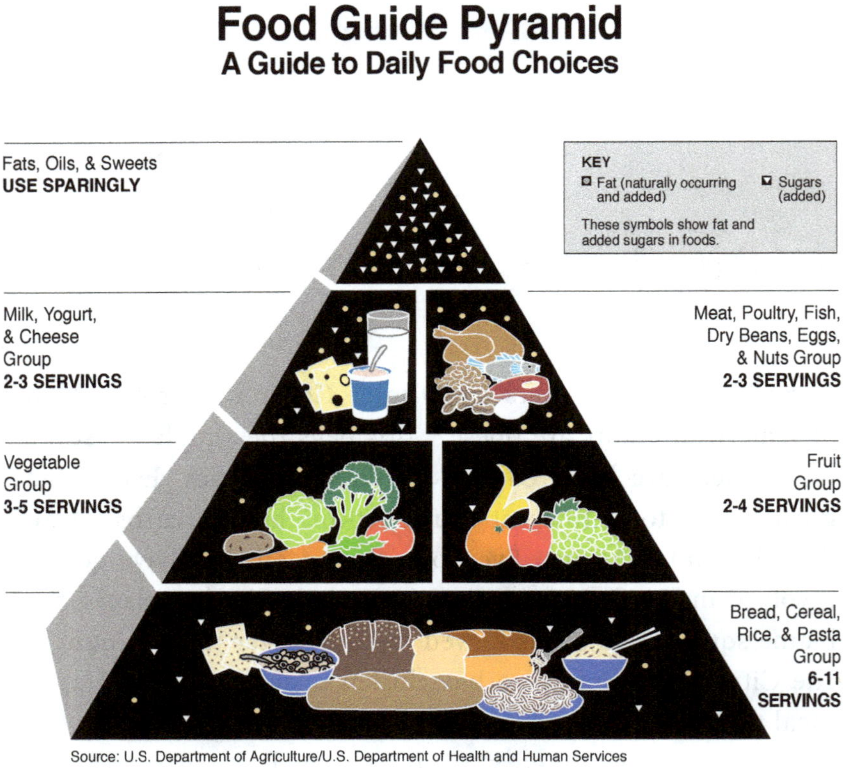

The Original Food Pyramid[3]

The interior of the *Pyramid* was piled high with breads, meats and vegetables so childishly drawn that they may actually be the historical precursor to clipart. In retrospect, the advice promoted by the *Pyramid* seems criminal. Without violating a single rule of the *Pyramid*, it is possible to eat as many servings of bread, white rice and pasta as all the other foods combined. That advice might be appropriate for a sumo wrestler. For the rest of us, it's a recipe for disaster.

We have countless friends who share our memories of elementary school classrooms plastered with USDA pyramids. We all have the same strange nostalgia for the bad advice of yesteryear.

This would be downright quaint if not for the fact that all of our memories are entirely manufactured.

The *USDA Food Pyramid* was first published in 1992. Any recollections from before that time, which include our own, could probably be used in a court of law to cast doubt on a person's sanity.

If you were born in the 1970s, this poster would have been hanging in your school lunchroom:

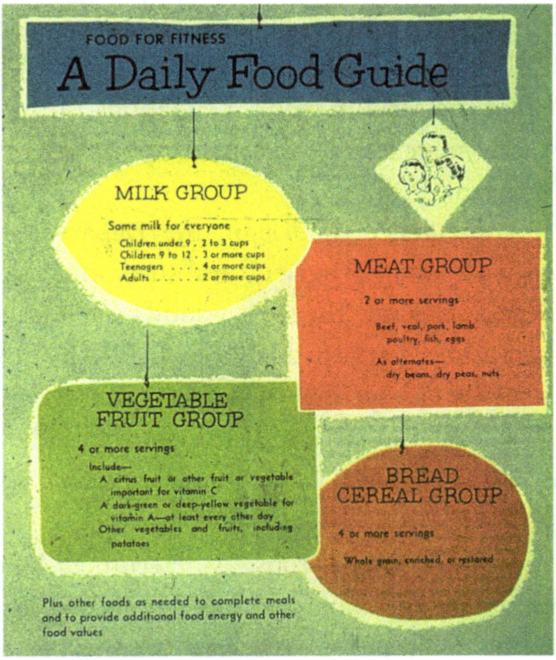

The Daily Food Guide[4]

The Daily Food Guide is slightly more reasonable when it comes to servings of bread, white rice and pasta. However, any potential caloric benefit of limiting these starches is undone by the recommendations that every single person drink a minimum of 300 calories of milk per day. *The Daily Food Guide* also took the outrageous position that a potato is fully equivalent to a serving of leafy green vegetables. As far as we are concerned, this is medical malpractice.

The one thing *The Daily Food Guide* and the *Food Pyramid* have in common is that both read as though they were designed not by scientists or nutritionists but rather by lobbyists from large agricultural companies. We are not conspiracy buffs. We believe that the moon landing took place on the actual moon and we reject the notion outright that the planet is being run by either a cabal of Jews or Reptile People.[5] It is not without a lot of forethought that we make the following accusation: it is far too convenient that the serving recommendations in the 1992 *Food Pyramid* exactly match the economic importance of the crops harvested that same year.

Either by coincidence or design, the Department of Commerce published a national agricultural survey for the same year the *Pyramid* was released. The survey shows the number of acres planted and bushels harvested nationwide.[6] Any five-year-old reading the survey can see that the largest crop in 1992 was corn, followed by wheat. The base of the *Pyramid*, with the largest number of recommended servings, is populated with cereal grains.

The next most important crops, as determined by the survey, are the fruits and vegetables that, amazingly, occupy the next level up in the *Pyramid*. Continuing toward the top of the *Pyramid*: we find meats and dairy products, which should come as no surprise, since chickens, beef cattle and dairy cows were the country's next most important agricultural products after fruits and vegetables.

While we have no hard evidence of undue political influence, we can safely surmise that if ConAgra or Monsanto had produced a Food Pyramid in 1992 designed to shift American's food tastes to match agricultural production, it would have been virtually identical to the one published by the USDA.

Roughly 2,600 years after Egyptians got out of the pyramid construction business, the USDA decided to join them. *MyPlate* was introduced to replace the Food Pyramid in 2011. According *The New York Times*, the U.S. Government spent over $2 million developing *MyPlate*, so it should come as no surprise that the design looks like the icon for the worst iPhone app ever.

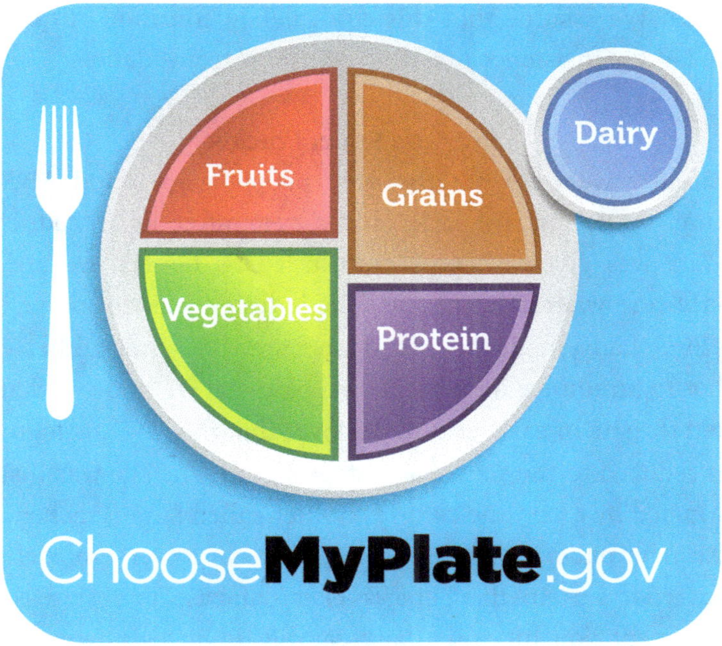

MyPlate[7]

At the *MyPlate* unveiling, First Lady Michelle Obama gave the least inspiring speech of any Obama in history: "When it comes to eating, what's more useful than a plate? What's more simple than a plate? The new design is a quick, simple reminder for all of us to be more mindful of the foods we are eating."[8]

Our reaction was, "That's supposed to be a plate? It looks more like a Trivial Pursuit playing piece being orbited by a racquetball."

The food recommendations behind *MyPlate* were shockingly similar to those of the Pyramid it replaced. The USDA still endorsed a diet containing quantities of grains and starches so large that their sheer bulk was likely to limit fresh fruits and vegetables. *MyPlate* continued the Pyramid's fairytale definition of "vegetable" in which a cup of chopped white potatoes is considered to be the nutritional equivalent to a cup of broccoli or spinach. We assume that this equivalency continued to be promoted at the insistence of a senior Senator from Idaho.

Enter the SuperTracker

Apparently we were not the only people who found *MyPlate* lacking. Sometime in 2012, only a year after its introduction, *MyPlate* was given a major facelift. To be honest, we are not exactly sure when it happened. The redesign was not publicized. The First Lady made no public appearances. They didn't even bother to announce it on their own blog. All we know is that we visited the site in early 2013 to discover that the *MyPlate* logo had been reduced to the size of a postage stamp. The site was instead dominated by an online calorie counter called SuperTracker.

The new pitch is simple: religiously record every morsel that passes your lips in the SuperTracker database and stop eating the moment you hit your daily calorie limit. This represents a monumental shift from the USDA's historical food group and serving-size-related recommendations. "Consuming fewer calories than expended will result in weight loss," the new SuperTracker explains. "This can be achieved over time by eating fewer calories, being more physically active or best of all, a combination of the two."[9]

The addition of SuperTracker represents a huge philosophical change. The USDA is now directly promoting the idea that calorie consumption drives both weight gain and loss.

While we agree with this philosophical shift, the actual advice given out by the SuperTracker system is highly suspect. SuperTracker's recommendations are so skewed towards grains and other starches that, if we were in charge, we would have named it Carb-O-Matic.

> **Fact:** Steven's customized, SuperTracker diet plan includes 10 slices of bread per day. Andrea weighs considerably less than Steven so her plan includes only nine slices of bread per day.

As advocates for the idea that it is possible to lose weight while continuing to drink alcohol, we accept that it is possible to cut calories while simultaneously eating 10 slices of bread a day. It merely requires eliminating enough other calories to make room. It can be done. We're just not sure why anyone would want to do it.

> **Fact:** Most commercial breads rings up between 80 and 100 calories per slice. White bread and wheat bread are not significantly different in this regard. So the USDA requirement that half Steven's slices come in the form of whole-grain bread makes little caloric difference. In other words, SuperTracker allows Steven between 800 and 1,000 calories a day from what they refer to as the "Grains Group."
>
> Allow us to put this into Drink Your Carbs perspective. A full bottle of wine totals between 600 and 650 calories. A pint of Guinness has 210 calories. A shot of tequila is around 70 calories. In order to match the calories in his bread allotment, Steven would need to

drink all of these. Sufficed to say, if Steven managed to drink these 1000 calories in a single evening, he would no longer be able to fulfill the Drink Your Carbs exercise requirement.

We freely acknowledge that one of the reasons Drink Your Carbs requires exercise is to place a natural limit on the amount of alcohol drinkers can imbibe. But we are, once again, getting ahead of ourselves. We will share our recommended alcohol consumption guidelines soon enough.

Steven's SuperTracker recommendations further allow "empty calories" of up to 459 per day. These calories are defined as, "Calories from food components such as added sugars and solid fats that provide little nutritional value." It is worth noting that these calories are on top of Steven's bread ration. This leaves roughly 1,500 calories—half of Steven's permitted 3,000 calories per day—left for healthy, nutritionally dense foods such as fruits, vegetables and unprocessed meats. In order to limit himself to only 1,500 nutritionally dense calories per day he would have to start skipping lunch.

Fact: There is no requirement that Steven eat his entire grain/bread allotment or that he consumes all of his permitted empty calories. He could choose to spend those calories elsewhere. This does not, however, make the USDA recommendations more reasonable.

Look at it this way: telling people they are allowed to consume 10 pieces of bread but should actually stop sooner is like printing "Contains Two Servings" on the label of a candy bar and expecting people to stop eating it halfway through.

We welcome the USDA's recent acknowledgement of the importance of calorie consumption. This is a huge step in the right direction toward a healthier diet and American populace. Hopefully the next few years will see recognition that simple carbs should be further reduced in favor of more nutritionally dense fare. Some day they may even figure out that the calories in alcohol are actually lower—and thus easier to offset—than in many of the foods they currently endorse. Until then, there will be Drink Your Carbs.

Three

The Drink Your Carbs Food Pyramid

Our friend's seven-year-old daughter refuses to draw heads on her figures. Give her a piece of paper and set of markers and she will create a colorful world of birds, clouds, trees and flowers. Cavorting among them, headless bodies dressed in elaborate costumes. It's less morbid than it sounds. The last step in her creative process is to sketch a teapot onto each set of empty shoulders.

"Have you ever heard of the artist Magritte?" Steven asked.

She shook her head no.

"I love your picture," Steven added. "But I have to ask, why is everyone in your drawing half human and half tea service?

"I'm no good at faces," she answered, "but I'm great at teapots."

We considered commissioning our friend's daughter to draw our Food Pyramid. It's a no-risk enterprise, we thought. It is not possible to do worse than the offerings from the USDA. A hoard of teapot zombies stumbling through a crudely drawn triangle would be a huge improvement over their recommendations that people consume more simple carbs.

The reason we didn't hire her—aside from the legal and accounting complexities of state and federally required payroll deductions from child laborers—is that we wanted more than just a better pyramid.

We wanted to prove that it's possible to communicate complex diet recommendations in a simple, graphical representation. More importantly, we wanted our pyramid to deliver, at a glance, a basic understanding of the Drink Your Carbs diet. We think we nailed it.

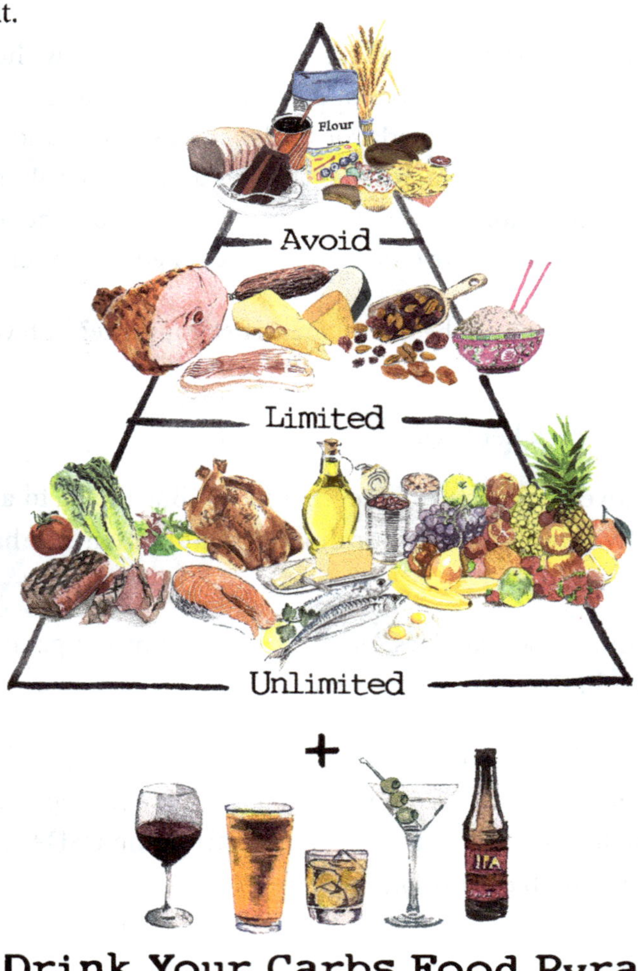

The Drink Your Carbs Food Pyramid

Four

Three Simple Steps to Get Started Now

In 2012, the Centers for Disease Control and Prevention published a brief under the dreary title, *Calories Consumed from Alcoholic Beverages by U.S. Adults, 2007–2010.*[1] Obviously, the first question that comes to mind is, why stop reporting numbers in 2010? The brief was released at the end of 2012. It can't possibly take two years to input survey data. If it does, we just found a new rallying cry for the grouchy old men who troll Internet news sites for opportunities to post angry comments about government inefficiency.

The conclusions of the brief were summed up in the first paragraph: "The U.S. adult population consumes an average of almost 100 calories per day from alcoholic beverages." The Internet exploded with editorials blaming alcohol for the obesity epidemic. The headline from *Men's Fitness* summed up the generally panicked tone: "The Cost of Drinking: 10 Extra Pounds of Fat a Year?"[2]

First, we think it's important to acknowledge that the CDC's 100 calorie number is an average and therefore meaningless. Allow us to offer the following analogy: if the population of America is split evenly, 50 percent men and 50 percent women, the average American has half a penis. Averaging drinkers and non-drinkers makes about as much sense. If you throw back a couple of drinks, you are very likely taking in more than 200 calories per day. Unless you also have a crappy diet and refuse to exercise, this is not a problem.

> **Fact:** As the CDC correctly notes, most Americans have a crappy diet and refuse to exercise. People take in too many calories compared to how few they burn. We disagree, however, with their solution. While the CDC encourages people to stop or reduce drinking, we recommend they instead continue drinking and address the real problem—their overall diet and exercise. We strongly believe that our solution is far more sustainable over the long term.

There is no secret to how Drink Your Carbs helps people to stay lean. The Drink Your Carbs Food List eliminates most sugars, starches and other high-carb foods. These foods tend to be high in calories while offering little nutritional value. Alcohol is allowed, but the calories we permit from alcohol consumption tend to be far less than the calories eliminated by the Food List. This works because alcohol is not nearly as caloric as people assume.

Allow Us to Offer a Few Examples:

- A single KFC extra-crispy chicken breast with no drink or sides packs 520 calories. This is half a glass short of drinking an entire bottle of wine.
- One regular-sized order of Outback Steakhouse's Aussie Cheese Fries is higher in calories than an entire 750ml bottle of Jack Daniel's whiskey. (We in no way endorse making this particular exchange.)

- Order a medium sized McDonald's Chocolate Shake and you will ingest 22-ounces of liquid with more calories than four pints of Guinness.
- A seemingly less extreme example is the "reduced fat" blueberry muffin from Dunkin' Donuts; it weighs in at 410 calories or just over two-thirds of a bottle of wine. Anyone who argues that it's okay to have a "low-fat" muffin but that alcohol is diet buster has never done the math.

We have been living and sharing this diet for nearly five years. We know for a fact that people are willing to exchange their empty calories for healthy meats, fresh fruit and vegetables if it means that they can reward themselves with a drink at the end of a day. In the words of our friend Dirk, who we will visit in more detail in Chapter Thirty, "Beyond health benefits, there is the psychological benefit of knowing I can still drink. I find it easier to stick to both working out and eating well knowing I can have a couple of drinks with dinner."

> **Fact:** Drink Your Carbs is designed to be a lifestyle. It can be worn like a pair of old, comfortable blue jeans. Most other diets are more akin to a medieval hairshirt.

Most people can successfully dive straight into Basic Drink Your Carbs. Some people, however, aren't ready to commit to a structure that requires a shopping list. We designed the Basic Food List to be comprehensive and flexible, but nonetheless we continually hear from people who are asking for simpler steps that can be implemented easily and quickly and without so much as a single trip to the supermarket.

Perhaps it's the flexibility that makes Food List difficult for some people. One friend told us, "There are too many choices here. I want something that doesn't require me to spend a ton of time thinking about it."

For her and for others who feel the same way, we have created Three Simple Steps.

These three steps are not as effective as Basic Drink Your Carbs, but they will get you 80 percent the way there. For most, this is more than enough guidance to start dropping weight. More importantly, once you fully implement these three steps, making the leap into Basic will be easy.

Step 1: Avoid All Deep-Fried Foods

In defense of deep-fried foods, they are likely to be the foods that allow humans to travel to Mars. The problem with deep-space travel is that each astronaut requires around 2000 calories per day to stay healthy. The trip to Mars will take roughly four years, two years there and two back. That adds up to a huge quantity of food that must be loaded alongside fuel, water, air and scientific equipment. The key to making the journey will be finding foods that are small in size but pack a wallop, calorie wise. In this one way, deep-frying is like a miracle. It adds an enormous number of calories while contributing little bulk. Of course, deep-fried foods also tend to be disgracefully low in vitamins, minerals and overall nutritional density. But that's a problem NASA scientists will have to solve for themselves. We can't do all their work for them.

If you're not preparing for a trip into deep space, deep-fried foods are more like a letter to Santa stating that all you want for Christmas is diabetes.[3]

Step 2: Avoid All Added Sugar and Other Sweeteners

This applies to food as well as drink.

In the rarified world of Drink Your Carbs, we refer to the no sweetened beverage restriction as the No Mixer Rule. It prohibits all sweet and sweetened beverages, including fruit juice. No Mixers is an exchange all drinkers must make in order to cut sufficient calories to both lose weight and continuing drinking alcohol.

No more sodas. No more orange juice. No simple syrup in your cocktails. No more schnapps or other sweet liquors. Fortunately, this is Drink Your Carbs: wine, beer and non-sweetened spirits are still very much allowed.

Step 3: Eat Nothing White

This rule should be treated as a guideline rather than a religious decree. The goal here is to eliminate simple starches from your diet. Unfortunately, nature lacks consistency. Most white foods, such as white bread, white rice and potatoes tend to be low in nutrition and high in calories.

Nature spawned a few white foods, such as cauliflower, egg whites and cooked chicken breast, which are the exact opposite. These white foods have high-nutritional density and should be part of a healthy weight-loss program. We considered adding an asterisk to "Eat nothing white." We considered changing the name of this rule to "Avoid all foods with a clown on the label."

Instead we will simply implore you to use common sense. Seriously, it's not that hard to figure out which white foods to eliminate. If you do get confused, we won't leave you hanging. First, check the label for artificial colors. Then look for more subtle signs. For example, the misspelling of "fruit" in Froot Loops should be a dead giveaway that the color cannot be trusted. The best policy is, if you're truly in doubt assume that the food you're contemplating is white and don't eat it. Choose something instead that is obviously and naturally colorful.

And we're not kidding about the clown on the label; those foods are definitely the kind of white you should never go near.

Five

The Basic Drink Your Carbs Diet

It is often said that one cannot "have one's cake and eat it too."

We say, "Forget the cake. It's rarely worth the calories. But do tell me what you have on tap behind the bar."

Basic Drink Your Carbs is our diet in its most simple form. Overhauling your diet on Basic is easy. We have done all of the work short of chewing your food. The Food List is the key. The Food List includes those foods that can be eaten all the time, those that should be eaten only on a limited basis and those that must be avoided altogether. The list is further broken into categories to make shopping easy. Some of your favorite foods are invariably in the "Avoid" category. This is the price you must to pay if you want to lose weight while continuing to drink alcohol.

Once you decide to embrace the Drink Your Carbs lifestyle, the first thing you should do is eliminate all non-Drink Your Carbs foods in your home. Everything that is labeled "Avoid" on the Food List has to go. This should be done even before you take the Food List to the grocery store for the first time. Donate your unopened cans to a local homeless shelter. Throw a party and serve the remainder to your friends and family. Do whatever it takes to get these foods out of your life before you start. The goal of this process is to make it more difficult to backtrack than it will be to move forward.

> **Fact:** We apply the same thinking to purging your home of unhealthy foods as Betty Ford employed with drugs and alcohol. Mrs. Ford insisted that, in order to start the healing process, her clients needed to distance themselves physically from the substances to which they were addicted. Without irony, we apply this same common-sense notion to the junk food in your kitchen.

Once you have completed the Drink Your Carbs equivalent of spring cleaning, you are ready to start. The Food List contains everything you need to put Drink Your Carbs to work in your life. Take it with you shopping. Use it as you read the menu in your favorite restaurant. Let the Food List be your guide and you will always find plenty of great options regardless of whether you're eating at home or eating out.

Tips for Using the Food List

The Food List does not contain every food item in existence. If it did, it would be roughly the size and weight of the 20-volume *Oxford English Dictionary.* You are certain to come across foods not on the list. Feel free to post any questions to our blog at drinkyourcarbs.com and we will try to reply quickly.

Alternatively, you can look for similar foods on the list to see where they fall. For example, we do not call out pattypan squash by name. We do, however, list zucchini under "Unlimited." Since pattypan is essentially UFO-shaped zucchini, you can safely assume it is also unlimited. Similarly, we do not explicitly prohibit funnel cakes by name, but between the sugar, the white flour and the deep fried preparation you should be able to figure out that they belong in "Avoid."

We have also included a list of food preparations to enjoy and to avoid. Just because zucchini is unlimited does not mean you are allowed to eat it breaded and deep-fried. How you prepare your food is as important as the foods you choose to eat.

Understanding the Categories: Unlimited, Limited and Avoid

Unlimited Foods

As long as you stick to Unlimited foods, you need not worry about portion size. Whereas some diets allow you to eat anything you want as long as the portion is small enough, Unlimited foods are truly unrestricted. There is no need to purchase a drug scale to weigh your portions. Or repurpose your drug scale if you're currently selling drugs. You can dress salads without the help of measuring spoons. You will never again drag your shirt cuffs through grease while trying to compare the size of your filet to that of your clenched fist. As long as you stick to Unlimited foods, the only constraint is that you stop eating when you feel full.

Limited Foods

The idea of limiting consumption causes confusion. We are convinced that somewhere out there, there's a thesaurus that lists "limited" as a synonym for "always." This is best explanation we have for why foods that are designated as Limited frequently become dietary staples.

Weight Watchers recently overhauled their entire point system to deal with the problem. Foods they intended to be limited became primary food groups for their membership. Weight Watchers solved the problem through hyperinflation. Certain foods now cost twice as many points within the system. The foods themselves are the same. All that changed was Weight Watcher's desire for their members to stop eating these foods so regularly.

> **Fact:** Supreme Court Justice Clarence Thomas was not the first porn hound appointed to the US Supreme Court. In 1964, Justice Potter Stewart spent hours and days in a tiny theater beneath the Court reviewing pornographic films. Justice Stewart did this under the pretense of doing research for an obscenity case, *Jacobellis v. Ohio.*
>
> No one knows exactly what Justice Stewart was doing during all of those lonely hours reviewing films; most historians presume that he was wearing his robes and taking notes in a dignified fashion. It is equally unknown whether there is still a grindhouse operating in the Court's basement. History recorded only that when Justice Stewart finally emerged in order to rule in favor of the pornographer he defined pornography as: "I know it when I see it."
>
> We have borrowed Justice Stewart's definition of pornography for own definition of Limited.

Defining what quantity of Limited foods is acceptable is extremely subjective. In the end, we all have to apply our own "I know it when I see it" test. We all have different weight-loss goals. We all have different caloric requirements in order to feel good and stay healthy as we diet. Deciding how much of any Limited food you should eat is more art than science. Our basic guideline is, if you are losing weight, continue eating the way you have been. If your weight loss slows, cut back on Limited foods. If you stop losing weight altogether, consider spending time in Austerity Mode where most Limited foods are banned altogether.

We included the Limited category because it offers more flexibility and variation than would be available if we instead put down blanket prohibitions. For example, most diets ban dried fruit. The usual justification is that dried fruit is higher in calories than fresh fruit. This is a fantastic reason, except that it's not true. A single dried peach is roughly equivalent in calories to a fresh peach, assuming the brand you have purchased contains no added sugar. The problem comes in the fact that it is far easier to eat a whole bag of dried peaches than a bag of fresh peaches.

For that reason, most diets ban dried fruit rather than trust dieters to control their intake. We have faith that you will behave like adults, so we have included dried fruit in Limited. This same belief holds true for all of the foods in this category.

> **Fact:** Steven eats no dried fruit because if he allowed himself to eat dried fruit he would eat an orchard's worth every single day.

Under no circumstances should you live off the foods on the Limited list. If you find yourself over-consuming one of these foods, cut it out. Again, the reason these foods are limited is that they are potential diet busters. It would not be difficult to eat an entire cup of roasted cashews, but doing so would add nearly 800 calories to your day. As long as they remain Limited, however, roasted cashews are a delicious, healthy snack.

Avoid

There are some foods you just don't eat.

> **Fact:** Losing weight while continuing to drink is as easy as pie—as long as you accept the fact that you can no longer eat pie.

Six

The Basic Drink Your Carbs Food List

UNLIMITED FOODS

Beverages

Beverages are fundamental to Drink Your Carbs. Beverages are the reason we developed the diet. We wanted to lose weight while continuing to drink alcohol. In order to accomplish this, however, some drinks had to go. Fortunately, there are plenty of great options left for your unlimited enjoyment.

Allowable beverages are as follows:

Alcoholic Beverages

Alcoholic Beverages and our "No Mixer" rule are discussed in depth in Chapter Fourteen. It is also worth reiterating that Drink Your Carbs requires exercise. Exercise is required for weight loss and overall health, but it also turns Drink Your Carbs into self-correcting system. If you cannot get out of bed in the morning to fully commit to your workout, you are drinking too much. It's time to dial it way back.

- Beer (Avoid obviously sweet beers and try your best to stick to lower-calorie beers.)
- Champagne and other sparkling wines (Avoid sweet sparkling

wines and champagne. Be aware that most of these wines contain small amounts of residual sugar. A good rule is to avoid Sec and Demi-Sec all together and ask for drier styles when ordering glasses or purchasing bottles. Brut, Extra Brut and Extra Dry are typically sensible choices.)
- Sake (No sweet sake.)
- Spirits (No sweet spirits, this includes spirits containing artificial sweeteners. Our reason for prohibiting artificial sweeteners can be found in Chapter Sixteen.)
- Wine—All red, white and rosé (No sweet wines.)

Non-Alcoholic Beverages

- Coffee (Iced, hot or room temperature. The best policy is: learn to like your coffee black. Do not add sugar or any artificial sweetener. If you must add milk, stick to non fat or skim.)
- Lemon, line and other citrus (We are not advocating drinking a tall glass of frozen, concentrated orange juice. In fact, juice is only allowed as a flavoring not as a primary beverage. Citrus should be fresh squeezed and unsweetened. Add only what is required to brighten to your drinks. Rose's Lime Juice does not count; if you check the ingredients you will find that Rose's is lime-scented high-fructose corn syrup.)
- Seltzer (Unsweetened. Cans and bottles labeled "Naturally Flavored" and "Zero Calories" are usually calorie free and unsweetened, but you should always check the ingredients to confirm that there are no artificial sweeteners.)
- Tea (All types, hot and iced, as long as they're unsweetened.)
- Water and sparkling water

Protein

All unsweetened meats and all varieties of eggs are allowed in unlimited quantity. All fish and other seafood are also unlimited.

We have yet to come across a fish, crustacean, bivalve or any other sea creature that is not perfect for Drink Your Carbs. This is not to say that scientists will not discover some creature living way down by the undersea vents that can swim yet has the basic body composition of a potato. Until this happens, the oceans are fair game. Consider everything from them to be unlimited.

> **Fact:** There is one exception to our blanket declaration that everything from the sea is unlimited. If it's on the endangered species list, it is not on Drink Your Carbs. There is no exception to this rule. If you really want to eat dugong or whale, lobby the U.S. Department of Fish and Wildlife to have them removed from the list. Until that happens, it's off the menu.
>
> There is one additional consideration, and it has nothing to do with carbs or calories. Some fish are dangerously high in mercury and other environmental pollutants. You don't have to take our word for it. The FDA has warned pregnant women and children not to eat certain fish.[1] If you think that ingesting toxins is more likely to give you superpowers than health problems, feel free to disregard the warning. For everyone else, we recommend checking out the Monterey Bay Aquarium's Seafood Watch program; they maintain a comprehensive list of both safe and sustainable seafood choices.[2]

We have divided protein into lean and high-fat proteins. Both categories are unlimited on Drink Your Carbs. However, if you want to lose weight a little faster, focus on lean meats. Lean meats are just as satisfying and can be significantly lower in calories. A simple rule to keep in mind is that grass-fed meats and wild-game meats tend to be leaner than grain and corn-fed animals.

Fact: We occasionally get angry letters detailing the treatment of industrially farmed animals and trying to convince us to stop eating and promoting meat. Our favorite letter included a photocopy of someone dressed as a cow, protesting outside of a McDonalds franchise.

We agree that industrial farming can be horrific. We just do not see that as a reason to quit meat altogether. Instead, we buy grass-fed meat from small family farms that do not use hormones or rely on feedlots. This is easy to do in San Francisco. It is markedly more difficult in other parts of the country.

Our best advice is that when you have the option of hormone-free, grass-fed meats, buy them. As more of us make this choice, more animals will be raised to these standards.

As for donning a cow suit and picketing a McDonalds, we support you 100 percent, although, for different reasons. A Big Mac contains 540 calories before you add a drink or fries. This is equivalent to nearly a full bottle of wine. To someone on Drink Your Carbs, the Big Mac is never worth it.

When you see a McDonalds, keep driving. And don't forget to wave to the kids out front in the cow suits. We're all on the same side.

Lean Protein

- Beef (Flank steak, roasts, lean ground beef, all grass-fed beef, and unsweetened beef jerky.)
- Buffalo
- Chicken Sausages (unsweetened)
- Deli Meats (unsweetened)

- Eggs (All types, from tiny quail to massive ostrich.)
- Fish and Other Seafood (All types including shellfish and roe.)
- Frog
- Game Meats (All types and cuts.)
- Goat
- Guinea Pig (Listed here for our Ecuadorian friends.)
- Insects (Keep this in mind while travelling or lost in the woods.)
- Organ Meats (All types. The spookier the better.)
- Pork Chops
- Pork Roast
- Pork Loin
- Poultry (All types and cuts, but do keep in mind that white meat is leaner.)
- Protein Powders (Egg, whey, pea, hemp and even brown rice-derived proteins are fine as long as they contain no added sweeteners.)
- Ostrich
- Rabbit
- Seitan (Yes, this is not meat. But it is a lean protein.)
- Sheep (Mutton)
- Snails
- Veal

Higher-Fat Proteins

- Bacon (unsweetened)
- Beef Ribs (Also called short ribs)
- Bologna
- Ham (unsweetened)
- Hotdogs (unsweetened)
- Jerky (unsweetened)
- Lamb

- Mortadella (Italian bologna)
- Pepperoni (unsweetened)
- Pork Ribs
- Pork Sausage (unsweetened)
- Prosciutto/Jamon Serrano/Jamon Iberico, etc. (Fancy, delicious cured pig parts.)
- Salami/Salumi
- Soy Proteins (tofu, tempeh, etc.)

Fats

- Butter
- Canola Oil
- Coconut Oil
- Flaxseed Oil
- Ghee
- Grape Seed Oil
- Lard and other Rendered Fats
- Nut Oils
- Almond Oil
- Cashew Oil
- Macadamia Nut Oil
- Pine Nut Oil
- Walnut Oil
- Olive Oil
- Peanut Oil
- Safflower Oil
- Sesame Oil
- Sunflower Oil

Fruit—All Fresh and Unsweetened Frozen, Including

- Apples (All varieties.)
- Apricots
- Apriums (If you haven't tried this hybrid, they are awesome.)

- Bananas
- Blackberries
- Blueberries
- Boysenberries
- Cherries
- Clementine
- Cranberries
- Figs
- Grapefruits
- Grapes
- Guavas
- Honeydew
- Kiwis
- Lemons
- Limes
- Loquat
- Lychee
- Mandarin Oranges
- Mangos
- Melons (All varieties.)
- Nectarines
- Oranges
- Papaya
- Passion Fruit
- Peaches
- Pears
- Persimmons
- Pineapple
- Plums
- Pluots (Another awesome hybrid.)
- Pomegranate
- Quince
- Pomelo

- Raspberries
- Strawberries
- Tangerines
- Watermelon
- Etc.—Pretty much anything that you can find raw in the produce section, go ahead and eat it.

Vegetables—All Fresh, Frozen and Unsweetened Canned

We love all vegetables, but we are particularly enamored with salad. We eat salad at nearly every meal. As far as we are concerned, a huge salad topped with some kind of protein is one of the great pleasures of being an omnivore.

Fifteen years ago, we visited the Galapagos Islands. Anyone who has studied Charles Darwin knows that these islands can have a strong and lasting impact on a young mind. Our trip lasted seven days. To this day, we show our affection for one another by performing the mating dance of the blue-footed booby.

When it comes to eating salad, we still channel our inner giant tortoise. The tortoises of the Galapagos grow to five feet in diameter and can weigh over 800 pounds. We never saw these giants in the wild, but at the Conservation Center we watched them devour leaves by the bushel. Their movements were slow and deliberate. Their focus was absolute. Imagine a vegetarian speed-eating contest filmed in Matrix Bullet Time.

The tortoises were unperturbed by visitors. In fact, they didn't give a rat's ass about the noise and the photographs as long as no one got between them and their leafy greens.

We serve our nightly salad from a bowl better sized for movie theater popcorn. As far as we are concerned—and we assure you that the tortoises agree—there is no such thing as too much salad.

- Asparagus
- Artichoke
- Arugula

- Avocados (No need to send us hate mail. We know avocado is technically a fruit. The problem is that if we categorize it under Fruit, no one would ever find it.)
- Bamboo Shoots
- Beans (All fresh varietals.)
- Beets and Beet Greens
- Broccoli
- Brussels Sprouts
- Cabbage
- Carrots
- Cauliflower
- Celery
- Chard
- Collards
- Corn (Whole, fresh kernels of corn on or off the cob. No popped, polenta, syrup or meal.)
- Cucumbers
- Dandelion Greens
- Eggplant
- Endive
- Garlic
- Ginger (fresh)
- Green Onion
- Herbs (All varieties. See Herbs and Spices.)
- Jerusalem Artichokes
- Kale
- Kholrabi
- Leeks
- Lettuce (All varieties including butter, iceberg, red leaf, romaine, etc.)
- Lemon Grass
- Mizuna
- Mushrooms (Dried and fresh.)

- Mustard Greens
- Okra
- Onions
- Parsnips
- Peas
- Peppers (Sweet and hot.)
- Radish
- Rhubarb
- Rutabagas
- Seaweed
- Shallots
- Soy Beans (edamame)
- Spaghetti Squash
- Spinach
- Summer Squash (zucchini, yellow, etc.)
- Tomatillos
- Tomatoes (Technically a fruit, but again most people don't know that.)
- Turnips
- Watercress
- Winter Squash (Acorn, Butternut, Pumpkin, etc.)
- Etc.

Non-Fat Dairy and Unsweetened Non-Dairy Milks

If you can tolerate dairy products—Andrea can, Steven cannot—they are a good source of protein. It is, however, possible to overdo it. Some dairy products, including high fat cheeses and yogurts, are calorically dense and way too easy to eat in large quantities. This is why most dairy is Limited on Drink Your Carbs. That said, we do allow non-fat dairy in unlimited quantities. Our reason is simple. Non-fat dairy is comparatively low in calories and high in protein.

To be clear: this recommendation has nothing to do with an irrational fear of fat. Most fats are unlimited on Drink Your Carbs, as are fatty meats. The reason high-fat dairy is Limited is due entirely to its calorie count. A tiny wedge of Brie has more calories than an entire cup of non-fat cottage cheese. By sticking to non-fat dairy, you get more food while consuming fewer calories.

We have also included a few dairy substitutes, as a nod to Steven and the rest of the dairy-impaired.

- Nonfat Cottage Cheese
- Nonfat Milk
- Plain, Non-Fat Yogurt (unsweetened) (If you are one of those people who cannot stand plain yogurt, try it with berries, fresh fruit and nuts, such as almonds or walnuts.)
- Unsweetened nut milks can be hard to find. We recommend that you make your own. The basic recipe is the same regardless of the nut used. We will use almonds for our example. Throw a handful of almonds and small cup of water into a really good blender. (Our favorite blenders are made by Vitamix and Blendtec). Hit "Start" and less than a minute later you should have thick, white almond milk. If it's too thin add more almonds. If it's too thick add water. You can find more complex recipes that require stirring and straining, but making nut milk really can be as simple as we describe.
- Almond Milk (unsweetened)
- Rice Milk (unsweetened)
- Soy Milk (unsweetened)
- Hemp Milk and Others (unsweetened)

Beans (Dried and Fresh)

Beans generate the most confusion of anything on the food list. We are aware that beans are high in carbs. They are also one of the best substitutes for rice, potatoes, etc. They are very filling, and, really, how many beans can you eat? If the answer is several cups in a sitting consider keeping these Limited. If not, enjoy.

- Azuki Beans
- Black Beans
- Black-Eyed Peas
- Broad Beans (fava beans)
- Cannellini Beans
- Chickpeas
- Great Northern Beans
- Green Beans
- Kidney Beans
- Lentils
- Mung Beans
- Pinto Beans
- Runner Beans
- Soybeans
- White Beans
- Etc.

Condiments, Herbs and Spices

All unsweetened condiments, herbs and spices are classified as unlimited. We strongly encourage their use. These are the ingredients that make a bland meal delicious. Herbs and spices have almost no calories and make everything taste better.

Branch out. Play. Seek out an ethnic grocery store or specialty spice shop. You will occasionally make awful, inedible mistakes, but you will also hit spectacular, towering home runs. One word of caution: beware of added sugar. You wouldn't expect to find high-fructose corn syrup in pickles, mayonnaise or mustard, but it's often there. Check the labels and you are good to go.

- Aioli (This is just a fancy word for mayonnaise.)
- Capers and Caper Berries
- Chili Paste (Asian style with or without garlic.)

- Dill Pickles (unsweetened)
- Harissa
- Mayonnaise (All types, including real, canola, olive-oil based and vegan "Nayonaise." Just make sure your choice is unsweetened. Miracle Whip, which we argue is not a type of mayonnaise at all, contains both corn syrup and sugar.)
- Mustard (unsweetened)
- Olives
- Pickled Vegetables (unsweetened, including cucumbers, beans, carrots, jalapeños, onions and others. Be on the lookout for fake color as well. Chances are, if it is dyed a primary color, it also contains sugar and/or corn syrup.)
- Relish (unsweetened)
- Salad Dressings (unsweetened)
- Salsa (Unsweetened. Read the labels carefully on fruit salsas. If they have no added sugar, they are okay.)
- Siracha (Our favorite hot sauce.)
- Sauerkraut
- Tartar Sauce (unsweetened)
- Tabasco, Chulula, Tapatio and other bottled vinegar/hot sauces. Just be sure to check for sugar.
- Vinegars (All varieties.)

Herbs and Spices

All unsweetened fresh and dried including:

- Allspice Berries
- Anise Seeds
- Annatto Seeds
- Asafetida
- Basil
- Bay Leaves
- Cacao Powder
- Cacao Nibs

- Caraway Seeds
- Cardamom
- Celery Seeds
- Chervil
- Chiles (All varieties.)
- Chives
- Cilantro
- Cinnamon
- Cloves
- Coriander Seeds
- Cumin Seeds
- Curry Leaves
- Dill Seeds
- Dill Weed
- Epazote
- Fennel Seed
- Galangal Root
- Garlic
- Ginger
- Hibiscus Flowers
- Horseradish Powder
- Juniper Berries
- Lavender
- Lemon Grass
- Lemon Verbena
- Lime Leaves, Kaffir
- Marjoram
- Mint Leaves
- Mustard Powder
- Mustard Seed
- Nutmeg
- Onion

- Oregano
- Paprika
- Parsley
- Peppercorns and Ground Pepper
- Rosemary
- Saffron
- Sage
- Salts
- Sesame Seeds
- Star Anise
- Tarragon
- Thyme
- Turmeric
- Vanilla Bean and Extract
- Wasabi Powder

LIMITED FOODS

As previously mentioned, defining Limited choices is more art than science. The key to Limited foods is that they should never comprise a full meal and they should never be a daily occurrence. Limited foods should be an occasional treat. If they stop feeling like something special, you are eating them too often. Limited foods are intended to provide variation and flexibility. If you find yourself living on any of these foods, you should eliminate it entirely. Alternately, you can move into Austerity Mode where most of these foods are forbidden.

Protein

Sweetened, processed meats are all Limited. We left them in Limited in spite of their sweeteners because they contain very little sugar and would be nearly impossible to fully eliminate. We recommend that you avoid buying sweetened meats to eat at home and instead save them for eating out. It will feel like a treat to order ham or maple bacon in your omelet, and not having these foods at home will help you keep them limited.

Examples of sweetened meats include:

- Bacon (Maple, honey, etc.)
- Beef/Buffalo Jerky
- Deli Meats
- Ham
- Pepperoni

Fats

After ridiculing diets that hold up certain foods as morally and nutritionally superior to others, we too are guilty of such prejudice. We categorize these fats as Limited because we believe that they are less healthy. That said, these highly processed oils are calorically similar to the so-called healthier oils listed under Unlimited. From a weight-loss perspective they are all about the same. Since this categorization is not about weight loss, but rather healthy eating, you should make your own choices. If you want to use highly processed fats or even trans fats in your cooking, we will not show up at your house to stop you. We just wanted you to be aware that we think there is a difference.

- Cottonseed Oil
- Palm Oil
- Margarine
- Shortening
- Soybean Oil
- Other Processed/Artificial Oils

Higher-Fat Dairy

All dairy, aside from non-fat dairy, is Limited. We do not distinguish low-fat from high-fat cheeses. The caloric difference between the low-fat and normal version of a cheese is often less than 10 calories per ounce. You are far better off eating the cheese you like and limiting the quantity.

- Cheese (All varieties except the kind that comes in a pressurized can. "Processed cheese foods" is not cheese. Based on the ingredients we would categorize it as a dessert topping.)
- Cream
- Milk (2% and above.)

Higher Calorie Alternative Milks

Most non-dairy milks contain a small amount of sugar to cut the bitterness of the nuts and other ingredients. These products are allowed in Limited quantity but we recommend reading the labels and trying to choose products with the least added sugar. As always, avoid flavored milks; premixed chocolate, strawberry, eggnog, etc. are a dead giveaway that a product contains too much sweetener and should be avoided.

- Coconut Milk (There is no added sugar in coconut milk, but one cup of the full fat variety contains over 500 calories. Use a splash of coconut milk in your coffee or use it to flavor dishes such as curry. If you want a glass of a milk-like-substance pick an alternative.)
- Soy Milk (sweetened)
- Almond Milk (sweetened)
- Rice Milk (sweetened)
- Other Sweetened Non-Dairy Milks

Nuts, Nut Butters and Dried Fruit (Unsweetened)

We love dried fruit and nuts. They are a great source of protein, healthy fats and fiber. More importantly, they taste great. We love them so much we could easily eat handful after handful. While that would be better for us than eating the same quantity of potato chips, it would still be a diet buster. Dried fruit and nuts pack a serious caloric punch. Enjoy them mightily, but eat them sparingly.

- Almonds and Almond Butter
- Brazil Nuts
- Cashews and Cashew Butter
- Chestnuts
- Coconut (unsweetened)
- Dried Fruits (All unsweetened varieties including dates, figs, apples, raisins, etc.)
- Hazel Nuts
- Fruit Jams and Jellies (unsweetened)
- Macadamia Nuts
- Peanuts/Peanut Butter (Yes, we know it's technically a legume. Feel free to create your own nerdy "legume" section in the margin if you feel strongly about it.)
- Pecans
- Pine Nuts
- Pistachios
- Pumpkin Seeds
- Sesame Seeds
- Sunflower Seeds
- Walnuts
- Etc.

Grains

In limited quantities, complex grains can be part of a healthy diet. The key here is to keep them limited. These foods are restricted for a reason. They are likely to add far more calories to a meal than would be added by any side dish of vegetables. That said, as long as they are consumed in reasonable quantities, they remain compatible with the Drink Your Carbs lifestyle.

Be careful not to overindulge on things like brown rice pasta or quinoa tortillas. In limited quantities these are fine, but it is very easy to overeat these foods. The same holds true for baked goods. Keep them as a treat rather than a staple. As with any food on the Limited list, if you can't control your quantities cut out grains entirely.

- Brown Rice, Wild Rice, Forbidden Rice
- Buckwheat
- Quinoa

Alternative Flours

If you want to bake or use flour in a recipe, stick to these higher protein alternatives. Just keep in mind that a gluten-free baguette, no matter how tasty, contains roughly the same number of calories as its glutinous counterpart, and sometimes more.

- Acorn Flour
- Almond Flour
- Bean Flours
- Buckwheat Flour
- Coconut Flour
- Quinoa Flour
- Tapioca Flour

AVOID THESE FOODS

Avoid is not as a strong a word as "prohibited." Food on the Avoid list will occasionally sneak into your diet. This is particularly true when you eat out. This is to be expected. Drink Your Carbs is a lifestyle not a religion. Avoid these foods as much as possible. Never bring them home from the grocery store. Never intentionally order a plate of them at a restaurant. This way, when they do sneak into your diet, they will do so in very small quantities.

> **Remember:** Ninety percent compliance with Drink Your Carbs is still an A on Major Morgan's Grading Scale (See Grading, Chapter Eleven).

Beverages

If you want to lose weight while continuing to drink alcohol, some beverages must be avoided:

- Gatorade and Other Sports Drinks, Including Coconut Water (You really don't need it unless you are running a marathon or something equivalent.)
- Juice (The only exception is a squeeze of citrus added to a dressing, recipe or cocktail for flavor.)
- Flavored Milk Drinks (Chocolate, strawberry-riffic, etc.)
- Mixers
- Sodas
- Diet Sodas (Our reason might surprise you, see Chapter Sixteen.)
- Sweet Liquors (Amaretto, Frangelico, Grand Marnier, etc.)
- Sweet Wines
- Vitamin Water and other flavored waters (Adding words like "Healthy," and "Vitamin-Enriched" to labels does nothing to change the fact that these are just flat sodas.)

High-Starch Vegetables

- Potatoes
- Sweet Potatoes
- Taro
- Yams

Grains and Flours

We don't avoid baked goods for a philosophical reason. Nor are we trying to torture ourselves like medieval monks or modern S&M

enthusiasts. We avoid these foods because they are obscenely high in calories. We simply cannot afford those calories if we also want to continue drinking.

- Barley
- Maize
- Millet
- Oats
- Potato Flour
- Rice Flour
- Rye
- Sorghum
- Wheat (This includes flour. This should be obvious, but we are continually surprised when we are told in restaurants that a dish contains "no wheat, only flour.")
- White Rice

Sugar and Other Sweeteners

Eliminating sugar and other sweeteners is by far the most difficult task most people face on Drink Your Carbs. Unfortunately, we can't make this any easier. These empty calories must be eliminated.

If you want to taste something sweet, eat fresh fruit. Fresh fruit is nature's candy and you can eat as much of it as you want. Also, keep this in mind when you are out to dinner: the Drink Your Carbs response to a dessert menu is, "My dessert is served in a glass."

Examples of sugars and sweeteners include:

- Agave Nectar
- Artificial Sweeteners (Our reasons might surprise you. See Chapter Sixteen.)
- Coconut Nectar
- Fruit Juice Concentrate

- Honey
- Maple Syrup
- Molasses
- Stevia
- Sugar (Brown, natural, powdered, white, etc.)

Condiments

All condiments containing sugar and other sweeteners including, but not limited to:

- Barbecue Sauce (Usually contains sugar.)
- Chutneys (Usually contains sugar.)
- Jams and Jellies (Sweetened. Pure fruit jams and jellies are limited.)
- Hoisin Sauce (Usually contains sugar.)
- Honey Mustard
- Ketchup (Usually contains sugar, or more likely, corn syrup.)
- Peanut Sauce (Usually contains sugar.)
- Sweet and Sour Sauce
- Sweet Pickles
- Teriyaki Sauce
- Thai Sweet Chili Sauce
- Etc.

PREPARATIONS

There is no shortage of experts recommending a raw food diet. To hear them tell it, heating your food instantly turns dinner into a toxic event analogous to Chernobyl. We'll let raw food guru Robert Ross speak for the entire raw food movement: "Heating food above 118 degrees [Fahrenheit] causes the chemical changes that create acidic toxins, including . . . carcinogens, mutagens and free-radicals . . ."[3]

We are more than a little skeptical. In fact, we're not convinced that a full-time raw diet is even good for you. Our skepticism is not based in scientific studies. It's based on the direct observation of people who work in raw food restaurants and profess to live a completely raw lifestyle. Members of the cult-of-raw are easy to spot because they tend to be thin and splotchy. And by thin, we are talking about the kind of thin that concerns New York models.

We recently ate at a raw-food restaurant in San Francisco. Our waitress was so thin and pale that even Kate Moss would have found herself whispering, "My God. Get that woman a piece of chicken."

If you plan on embracing the raw food lifestyle, you don't have to worry about preparations. All of your "cooking" will be done in a blender and a food dehydrator.

For those of us who still plan to cook some meals, we offer the following guidance on preparations: this list is designed to steer you away from preparation methods which turn otherwise low-calorie, healthy foods into calorie bombs. This list is particularly useful for eating out. Consider it a guide for translating the hyperbole that has become standard menu fare.

Unlimited

- Baked
- Barbequed
- Blanched
- Boiled
- Braised
- Broiled
- Chopped
- Cured
- Dried/Dehydrated
- Grilled
- Microwaved
- Pickled
- Poached

- Pureed
- Raw
- Roasted
- Rotisserie Cooked
- Sautéed in Oil, Water or Stock
- Slow Cooked
- Smoked
- Sous-Vide (Slow cooked in water while sealed in a pouch. Delicious.)
- Steamed
- Stewed
- Stir Fried (As in, not deep fried.)

Avoid

- Breaded
- Candied (As in "candied walnuts.")
- Chicken Fried
- Cream Sauced
- Crispy (This is generally a euphemism for "fried," but not always. We have seen it applied to foods that are Drink Your Cars friendly, such as baked in a hot oven and/or coated with nuts. At a minimum, the term "crispy" requires an extensive interrogation of the wait staff.)
- Deep-Fried
- Encrusted (Fancy for breaded.)
- Glazed (Almost always sweet.)

Visit drinkyourcarbs.com to download a free copy of the Condensed Food List. It contains every food, drink and condiment in the Food List without any commentary. Hopefully, it will carry you through to the day that we stop procrastinating and build a Drink Your Carbs app.

Seven

Austerity Mode

Austerity Mode can best be described as Drink Your Carbs on steroids. Or, if you are a professional cyclist and the mere mention of steroids triggers a panic attack, think of Austerity Mode as Basic Drink Your Carbs with all of the fun foods removed.

Basic Drink Your Carbs includes plenty of healthy carbohydrates, including an allowance for limited quantities of healthy starches such as brown rice and quinoa. In Austerity Mode, these foods are eliminated and virtually all carbohydrates come from fruits and vegetables. This is not to say that Austerity Mode turns Drink Your Carbs into a traditional low-carb diet. Austerity Mode still allows plenty of foods banned by the low-carb gurus. More importantly, Austerity Mode continues to allow for the consumption of alcohol. This alone distinguishes it from every other low-carb diet we have seen.

Fact: The difference between Basic Drink Your Carbs and Austerity Mode may seem trivial. Trust us: these differences have an enormous impact in what you're consuming. We recently spent a week in Austerity Mode and even for us it was a struggle. We were hungry the entire time. We would eat. Twenty minutes later we're desperate for a snack. As children, we read *The Very Hungry Caterpillar* but only after that week did we fully understand his manic food issues.

Here's the upside—Austerity Mode accelerates weight loss. By eliminating most of the remaining sugars and starches left in the Basic Drink Your Carbs diet, Austerity Mode further restricts calories. Assuming your exercise and alcohol consumption remain unchanged, the results will be predictable—and the weight loss will be dramatic. However, the increased pace of weight loss is not the only reason to spend time in Austerity Mode. There are numerous reasons that Austerity Mode is an invaluable part of the Drink Your Carbs dietary toolkit:

Faster Weight Loss

The most obvious reason has already been mentioned. If you want to lose a few pounds fast, Austerity Mode is the way to do it. Basic Drink Your Carbs, if followed consistently, will lean you down to a healthy weight. However, the weight loss tends to be slow and consistent. This is not a bad thing, as diets designed for fast weight loss tend to be difficult to maintain and are often followed by subsequent weight gain. But there are times when we want to see faster results. Whether it is for an upcoming competition, event or a fast-approaching high school reunion, sometimes the pace of weight loss matters. Austerity Mode is the answer.

Chasing the Perfect Bikini/Speedo Body

Weight loss on Basic Drink Your Carbs will eventually level off. Your caloric requirements go down as you lose weight. The less body mass you have to maintain, the fewer calories you need to maintain it. Eventually, we all come to a point where our calories and exercise fall into balance. Weight loss stops and maintenance begins. Drink Your Carbs is designed so that this leveling off will occur at a healthy, sustainable weight.

Anyone who has dieted will tell you that there is a difference between being lean and healthy and turning heads in a bikini or Speedo. Keep in mind that there appear to be no additional health benefits from achieving this next level of lean. The only reason to pursue it is for pure aesthetics.

The perfect bikini/Speedo body is not easy to attain. The older you are, the harder it is to get. The discipline required is enormous. You might have to spend more time in Austerity Mode than not. But if you want to pursue this goal, Austerity Mode is our tool to get you there.

> **Fact:** Bikinis are fashionable worldwide but the same cannot be said for the Speedo. Outside of platform diving and Michael Phelps' closet, the Speedo is much maligned. If you want one, you'll probably need to shop for it in a specialty store for either professional swimmers or Eastern Europeans.
>
> If you choose to wear a Speedo, expect your friends to refer to it by unflattering nicknames, such as "man panties," the "banana hammock" or the "budgie smuggler"—ask an Australian if you want to know what a budgie is. We strongly disagree with all of this negativity. If you spend the time in Austerity Mode to get yourself into shape to wear it, we say ignore these self-appointed fashionistas. Strut your stuff like a bird in the full plumage of mating season. You have earned the right.

Advance Preparation for an Epic Event or Weekend

This simple notion may be the most revolutionary idea in Drink Your Carbs. We are shocked not to have come across it in other diets. This idea is so blindingly obvious that it really should be part of every diet plan. As far as we know, this is a Drink Your Carbs exclusive.

We will further explore this idea in Chapter Ten, How to Cheat on Your Diet. We are discussing this strategy here as well because it really is useful.

While every major diet has a section or chapter titled "How to Stay on Your Diet While on Vacation," only Drink Your Carbs allows you to prepare in advance for a guilt-free holiday.

We all have events on our calendars that we know will blow our diets. Perhaps you are planning to visit relatives who don't share your Drink Your Carbs obsession. You might be taking a cruise, complete with a midnight chocolate buffet that you know you probably can't—and won't—avoid. A wedding, charity dinner or office party is equally likely to knock you off Drink Your Carbs. All of these events have one thing in common: they are scheduled well in advance. You have plenty of notice. Austerity Mode is the strategy that will help you prepare.

Before you embark on a vacation or attend an event where staying on Drink Your Carbs will be difficult, go into Austerity Mode. The idea is to build up a calorie deficit in advance of the event. That way you can enjoy yourself without guilt or regret.

> **Fact:** We acknowledge expert opinions are mixed on banking calories from one day to the next. Some claim that it works in a limited way. Others believe that dieters simply lose weight when cutting calories and regain that weight later when more calories are consumed. From our perspective, it makes no difference which group turns out to be correct. The end result is the same. If you have lost weight in advance of a cheat, you have earned a cushion and can enjoy yourself more freely.

The bigger the cheat is likely to be, the more time you need to spend in Austerity Mode. Planning for a blowout Christmas party requires spending a few days in Austerity Mode beforehand. The cruise would take longer. Before embarking on that kind of trip, we would go Austerity Mode for a couple of weeks. In exchange, we would allow ourselves to enjoy the vacation without beating ourselves up every time we are handed a complimentary sickly sweet cocktail.

Deciding how long to prepare for a planned cheat is more art than science. We suggest you err on the side of over-preparing. There is no downside; if you go into Austerity Mode for longer than needed you might lose a little extra weight.

Dietary Reset Button

Just like everyone else, we occasionally find ourselves drifting away from our diet. This typically happens when we have family in town or otherwise find ourselves eating out more often than we eat in. At first, we cheat in small ways, snagging a few French fries off a nearby plate. With each cheat we grow bolder. Eventually, we find ourselves justifying fish and chips, or even sipping on a cocktail sweet enough to qualify it as dessert. It's embarrassing to admit how quickly small cheats snowball into bigger ones. Suddenly we are no longer even close to adhering to Drink Your Carbs.

A week in Austerity Mode acts as a diet reset. It is not easy, but seven days is enough to kill our sugar cravings and rededicate us to the Drink Your Carbs lifestyle.

Eight

The Austerity Mode Food List

Austerity Mode eliminates nearly all the remaining sugars and starches left in Basic Drink Your Carbs. Sweet Protein, Alternative Flours and Limited Grains are now to be avoided. Beans are now Limited because, while they are an excellent source of very filling fiber, they are also high in carbohydrates. All other categories remain the same.

Do not expect Austerity Mode to be easy. Going cold turkey on sugar and simple carbohydrates—even if they are already at a very low level in your diet—is akin to trying to kick a heroin habit without methadone or so much as a single therapy session. It brings all the symptoms associated with addiction withdrawal. (We were planning to list the symptoms here, but instead we will just recommend that you rent *Sid and Nancy*.)

The last time we spent a week in Austerity Mode, Steven found himself standing in Walgreens staring longingly at the snacks in the junk food aisle. And by snacks, we're talking about plastic-wrapped, artificially flavored "baked goods." For the record, the reason they wrap these foods in plastic has nothing to do with preserving freshness; it is to keep them from gathering dust. There is no need to keep them fresh since they are injected with all manner of synthetic ingredients to ensure that they age without any noticeable degradation. They are like Cher; anything that can be done is being done to ensure their exterior hull retains its alluring shape. When foods this bad look good, you know that you are having serious carb cravings.

> **Fact:** Our friend Elliott once spent two hours during a nasty winter storm tearing apart dresser drawers, searching under his car seats and even sifting through ashtrays in a futile attempt to find a cigarette that might have somehow been overlooked. In the end, he emptied the tobacco out of every stubbed out butt he could find and smoked them in a pipe made of tinfoil.
>
> As far as we're concerned people who consume pre-packaged baked goods with a shelf life approaching infinite should view themselves as no different from Elliott. They are not seeking a pleasurable experience. They are looking for a fix.

Stay disciplined. This process is not easy, but it does get easier. As each day passes, the cravings will diminish. For most people, in about a week they will vanish altogether.

AVOID

Sweetened Protein

These meats often contain very little sugar or other sweeteners. Nonetheless, they are to be avoided in Austerity Mode. The only exception is for products that contain absolutely no added sweeteners. They do exist, but they are hard to find.

- Beef/Buffalo Jerky (sweetened)
- Deli Meats (sweetened)
- Bacon (sweetened)

- Ham (sweetened)
- Pepperoni (sweetened)

Grains

There is no question that grains add far more calories to a meal than a side dish of vegetables. While we believe that limited quantities of these complex carbohydrates should be part of a healthy diet, the following grains are to be avoided in Austerity Mode:

- Brown Rice, Wild Rice, Forbidden Rice, etc.
- Buckwheat
- Quinoa

Alternative Flours

Avoid all alternative flours. You can resume your occasional baking when you get back to Basic Drink Your Carbs.

- Acorn Flour
- Almond Flour
- Bean Flours
- Buckwheat Flour
- Coconut Flour
- Quinoa Flour
- Tapioca Flour

LIMITED

Beans (Dried and Fresh)

- Azuki Beans
- Black Beans
- Black-Eyed Peas
- Broad Beans (Fava Beans)
- Cannellini Beans
- Chickpeas

- Great Northern Beans
- Green Beans
- Kidney Beans
- Lentils
- Mung Beans
- Pinto Beans
- Runner Beans
- Soybeans
- White Beans
- Etc.

Nine

Nightmare Mode

Nightmare Mode is Austerity Mode without booze. Nightmare Mode is the only time on Drink Your Carbs that you are not allowed to drink.

The Nightmare Mode Food List is the same the Austerity Mode Food List, but Nightmare Mode further eliminates all alcohol consumption.

As far as we are concerned, Nightmare Mode barely qualifies as Drink Your Carbs. It's like observing Meatless Monday on the Atkins diet. It's an across-the-board revision so extreme that it's arguable you are no longer on the diet at all. That said, we have several reasons for keeping it around:

Even Faster Weight Loss

There is no question that eliminating alcohol accelerates weight loss beyond what is possible in Basic Drink Your Carbs or even Austerity Mode. There are calories in alcohol. Eliminate these calories and weight falls off. If you have a tight deadline by which you must fit into tight pants, Nightmare Mode may be your only option.

This is not Drink Your Carbs; this is a panic button. Use only in emergencies.

Penance

While it's rare, we occasionally drink too much and skip a morning workout. Exercise is required on Drink Your Carbs, and, as far as we are concerned, exercise keeps our drinking in check. We temper our drinking with the knowledge that in the morning we will be in the gym doing something painful. However, in spite of our best efforts, we occasionally overdo it.

Depending on the severity of our transgression, we do penance of a few days to a week in Nightmare Mode. This is not a requirement of Drink Your Carbs. We have chosen this punishment because the ever-present threat of Nightmare Mode keeps us, for the most part, under control.

The next time your inner Charlie Sheen gets the best of you and trashes your diet like a Vegas hotel room, give Nightmare Mode a try. It is a fast and effective way to get you back on track.

A Check to Make Sure Our Drinking is Still Healthy Drinking

Alcohol can be addictive. We use Nightmare Mode to keep ourselves in check. We spend one week in Nightmare Mode roughly every three months. We have a friend who goes into Nightmare Mode for one month out of every year. We do this to make certain that we are still in control of our alcohol consumption.

For us, not drinking for a week is not particularly difficult. We simply remind ourselves that we could live for seven days without food; giving up booze for that long is no big deal.

The 30-Day Nightmare Mode Experiment

Last year we carried out an experiment and spent 30 days in Nightmare Mode. Normally, we would have used rats for this experiment, but we find ourselves to be cheaper and easier to care for. In the past, we had mostly used Nightmare Mode for self-flagellation. Our 30-day Nightmare Mode experiment was different. We were not punishing ourselves. We did it because we were curious how it would make us feel. How would it affect our sleep, our workouts and overall energy levels?

We can now say in no uncertain terms that 30 days in Nightmare Mode is completely overrated. Our sleep patterns did not change. We felt no more energetic in our workouts than we did while drinking.

> **Fact:** Steven insists that the 30-day Nightmare Mode challenge is like volunteering to spend a month in a cage at Guantanamo. Andrea thinks that this is way overstated.
>
> Andrea says it's more like spending 30 days on a flight to nowhere, in a middle seat, in the back of the plane, next to a crying child and with a toddler endlessly kicking her chair from behind. Oddly, Steven finds this too extreme.

What surprised us most on our extended journey into Nightmare Mode was that eating out was easier than cooking at home. Not having a drink with dinner at a restaurant isn't all that noticeable.

When we went out, we ordered iced tea or sparkling water without feeling particularly deprived. When we stayed at home, however, not opening a bottle of wine or uncapping a beer was painful. One night we grilled beautiful grass-fed porterhouse steaks. We served them along side our favorite side dish, Perfect Kale—the recipe can be found in Chapter Thirty Two. A glass of red wine or a dark beer would have perfectly balanced the meal.

We stayed strong and drank only water, but we couldn't shake the feeling that something was missing. It was like listening to the Rolling Stones with the bass turned all the way down.

On the plus side, we both lost a couple of pounds. We have always maintained that cutting out the calories in alcohol speeds up weight loss and we experienced that firsthand. It also turns out that eating out is far less expensive for non-drinkers. Every time we ventured out, the bill was half the usual price.

We completed the experiment, but we certainly don't recommend it to anyone else. The whole point of Drink Your Carbs is that if you eat well and exercise you can reward yourself with a drink at the end of the day. Take that away and most of the joy of this diet goes with it.

Ten

How to Cheat on Your Diet

Fact: We live in a time of plenty. This is a good thing. Yes, it is true that statistically most of us will end up blind and wheelchair-bound from Type-2 Diabetes, but the alternative is still worse. If you don't believe us, go ask your grandparents about the Great Depression.

One side effect of living in a time of plenty is that temptation is everywhere. Unless you possess super-human will power, you will occasionally fall off of your diet. Rather than chastise or embarrass you, we have developed strategies to help you cheat. It is not that we encourage cheating. We don't. Cheating on Drink Your Carbs will slow or stop your weight loss. We'd prefer if you never strayed from the Food List and our exercise recommendations. We acknowledge, however, that cheating happens and our goal is to help you contain the damage.

There are two ways people cheat on their diet: planned and unplanned cheating. This also is true for cheating on spouses, exams and in poker games, but that is outside of our current scope.

Unplanned Cheating

Unplanned Cheating means that you started the day with the best of intentions, but somehow found yourself eating half a box of Krispy Kreme doughnuts. This is usually a problem of availability.

You might never buy this crap, but someone else brings the box of doughnuts to a meeting and sets it on the table in front of you. Nearly a whole day's worth of calories vanish into your belly before you even realize what you are doing.

Sometimes you lay waste to your diet because a restaurant's special is an absolute favorite. Or you arrive at a bar after work to discover that your friends have taken the liberty of ordering pitchers of sickly sweet margarita and the All-the-Fried-Food-You-Can-Hold-Down Pu Pu platter. The fact is that we all occasionally fall short of our best intentions.

> **Fact:** The key to overcoming an unplanned cheat is not to beat yourself up about it. Guilt and self-loathing burn surprisingly few calories, so there is little advantage to dwelling on your transgression.

It is also not worth trying to burn all of those extra calories in a single, extended session at the gym. You'll need to run 11 miles to burn off the 1,400 calories packed into six glazed donuts. If you're training for a half marathon, it might be an option. Otherwise, you risk hurting yourself by attempting a level of exercise for which your body simply is not ready. Burning it all off at once isn't realistic most of the time.

Nor is shame starving. It is neither healthy nor effective to starve yourself in penance. Though this is an extremely common response to an unplanned cheat, it has exactly the opposite effect than desired. Starvation leaves you ravenously hungry, which makes you more likely to cheat on your diet again. If you allow yourself to get hungry enough, your evolutionary conditioning takes over. You will inevitably find yourself gorging on the nearest available food, whatever that food may be. The odds are that the nearest available food is as bad for you or worse than the unplanned cheat which started the cycle.

Fact: The starve-and-binge cycle—appallingly common among dieters—is the same strategy sumo wrestlers use to bulk up for competition.

Some researchers claim that this cycle shocks the body's metabolism into slowing down and storing more weight than it would have if the same calories were spread evenly over a day. Other researchers argue that starving and binging is all about calories consumed; they believe that the cycle simply allows people to eat more than would be possible without the periods of starvation in between. Differences of findings aside, they all conclude that starving yourself is only a good strategy if you are actively trying to pack on pounds.

The best way to overcome an unplanned cheat is simply move on. Acknowledge that it happened and go back to strict Drink Your Carbs. If you are really worried that you have slowed your weight loss, spend a few days in Austerity Mode. Either way, the key to getting through an unplanned cheat is to get back on your diet as quickly as possible.

Planned Cheating

Most diets spend multiple chapters on unplanned cheating, how to avoid it and how to properly flagellate yourself afterwards. For some reason, planned cheating is completely off their radar, even though it is universal to all dieters. This idea is so blindingly obvious that we fully expect every major diet to steal it and claim it as their own invention. It is just a matter of time until we see the headline and think, like David Bowie hearing *Ice Ice Baby* for the first time, "that sounds really familiar."

When you visit relatives, you give up significant control over your food choices. Unless you are lucky enough to be visiting relatives who also live the Drink Your Carbs lifestyle, they will feed you whatever it is that they normally eat. In most cases, especially if they are American, they eat garbage and lots of it.

We can tell you with absolute certainty that next Thanksgiving everything served at Steven's childhood home will be either starch, deep-fried, or, more commonly, deep-fried starch.

Knowing this a full year in advance leaves us with two choices: we can wait until Thanksgiving, swearing to ourselves that we will stick to dry turkey and over-steamed green beans, then find ourselves in the middle of an unplanned cheat or we can acknowledge up front that we are going to fall off of our diet for a few days.

The advantage to the second path is that it enables us to plan. A few days before Thanksgiving, we shift into Austerity Mode. We are incredibly strict with our diets. We sometimes even add a few extra sessions at the gym. Before the first family meal is served, we have banked enough calories that we can approach the holiday guilt-free.

Everyone should have planned cheats on their calendar coinciding with events where you just won't be able to stick to your diet. A birthday is an obvious planned cheat day. A dinner with your boss or co-workers is likely to be a cheat meal. It is difficult, if not impossible, to keep to strict Drink Your Carbs on Christmas, Valentine's Day or the Fourth of July. This is equally true of weddings, Bar Mitzvahs, Baptisms and even funerals.

Holidays, life-cycle events and vacations all share one thing—the possibility of advance planning. The moment you agree to attend, you know that at best your diet will slip a little, and at worst your caloric intake will rival that of a veal calf. This knowledge allows you to perform the Drink Your Carbs equivalent to the Polio booster and immunize yourself by going into Austerity Mode to build up a calorie deficit before any cheating takes place.

The key to successful planned cheating is to figure out the extent of your upcoming calorie splurge. A birthday blowout can easily be prepared for with a few days in Austerity Mode. A week-long culinary tour of Tuscany or a deep-fried weekend in New Orleans will take longer. Before embarking on that kind of trip, we would go strict Austerity for at least a few weeks.

Try to be realistic and prepare sufficiently so that you can enjoy your planned cheat without any of the shame or regret that ordinarily accompanies unplanned cheats. Remember that if you go into Austerity Mode for longer than needed, the only side effect is that you might lose a little extra weight.

Eleven

Grading Your Performance

How strict is strict enough for Drink Your Carbs?

We grade our own compliance using the same letter system used by the meanest, toughest teacher in the world. That teacher taught at our middle school. She was a small woman with a fair complexion and sandy blonde hair. But her mild-mannered appearance fooled no one. She ruled her classroom with an iron fist. She had no first name. In her presence, she was Mrs. Morgan. Outside of her presence, everyone referred to her as "Major Morgan."

Major Morgan cut no slack and tolerated no dissent. Everyone who knew her feared her. We would occasionally find a student who had just left Major Morgan's class crying in the hallway. Of course, if you survived her class with a decent grade you were, from that day forward, impossible to intimidate. Every other teacher you might come across and every other class you might attend seemed easy by comparison.

The purpose of this exercise is not to inspire guilt. The goal here is to do an honest evaluation of your adherence to Drink Your Carbs.

We understand that 100 percent compliance is rare. Most of us do not prepare all of our own meals so we are often faced with choices that are less than ideal. The reason to evaluate your own performance continually is to keep non-compliance to a minimum. Regular grading allows you to make corrections before an occasional cheat becomes a permanent habit, before one bad meal becomes your new baseline.

Major Morgan issued a weekly pop quiz. At the time, we assumed she did this out of spite. As adults, we now understand that Major Morgan wanted us to regularly check our performance so that we would be able to react quickly if it began to degrade. We suggest you adopt Major Morgan's model and grade yourself weekly.

When you grade your own compliance, feel free to channel an inner Major Morgan if you do not have a teacher of your own to draw upon.

Major Morgan's Grading Scale

90 to 100% compliance is an A.

Congratulations. Take yourself out for a drink.

80 to 90% compliance is a B.

Not bad. You are probably losing weight, but you could be losing weight faster.

Below 80% is a failing grade. (We warned you that Major Morgan was a hard ass.)

You are not on Drink Your Carbs. If you're losing weight while adhering to the diet less than 80 percent of the time, your pre-Drink Your Carbs diet must have been truly horrific. But if you are losing weight, we recommend that you continue doing whatever it is that you are doing, even if it isn't technically Drink Your Carbs. When you stop losing weight, try increasing your compliance. We think you'll be happy with the results.

Remember: Major Morgan did not grade on a curve. If all of your friends are failing, it won't boost your grade. Everyone is graded individually on his or her own performance. In this case, some children will be left behind.

Twelve

Maintenance

Most diets give the false impression that weight maintenance is a simple task. They assure you that, with a few modifications to your lifestyle, your weight will not fluctuate as long as you adhere to their formula.

Anyone who has ever dieted and then tried to maintain his or her target weight knows that it's not easy. No matter how hard we fight it, our weight fluctuates. Perhaps work gets busy and exercise falls to the wayside for a week or two. A friend or relative comes into town and we find ourselves eating out every meal for five days in a row. A simple formula fails in a complex system, and everyday life is far more complex than most diet plans are willing to admit. In the most extreme cases, these formulas fail so spectacularly that the dieter regains all of their lost weight and more.

There's no secret formula for weight maintenance. Instead, we designed Drink Your Carbs to be flexible enough to adapt to a constantly changing lifestyle.

First, you need to determine your target weight. Some people have an immediate objective in mind, but it helps to check with a professional. A doctor or personal trainer will be able to help you identify a healthy range. At first, your goal should be the upper end of that range. Over time, as your body grows accustomed to your new weight, feel free to dial that number downward.

The U.S. Department of Health and Human Services recommends using Body Mass Index, or BMI, to figure out your goal weight. They have online charts which, by lining up your height and weight, will tell you your current and ideal body mass. We don't care that the BMI scale is endorsed by hundreds of government scientists. We think the system sucks.

Case Study in the Failure of the Body Mass Index: We have a close friend who epitomizes our objection to the BMI scale. This friend is very athletic. He works out five days a week in the gym. On weekends he goes for long bike rides, dragging himself and his road bike over mountain passes high above Denver, Colorado. His body fat hovers around 12 percent. He is also seriously built; his muscles would still be visible if you dressed him in a burka. By all definitions, he is super fit. He also happens to be 5' 4" and, according to the BMI scale, he is morbidly obese. This is just plain stupid.

Apparently, these failures are not uncommon for anyone who is short, tall or carries a lot of muscle mass. Until BMI is updated to take people like our friend into account, we recommend that you ask your doctor or a personal trainer at your gym to help you calculate your ideal weight. They will give you a far more accurate answer based on your body type and muscle mass.

Once your goal is reached, you need to monitor your weight regularly to see if you are still losing, gaining or holding steady. Your weight will fluctuate. There is no such thing as keeping your weight steady. Anyone who claims otherwise has never stepped on a scale twice in the same day. The key to maintenance is to keep your fluctuations within a reasonable range.

Strive to keep your weight within a three-pound range. If you fall three pounds below your goal weight, you can relax your diet a bit. If you find yourself three pounds above your goal weight, it is time to increase your adherence to Drink Your Carbs, or even consider spending time in Austerity Mode. The sooner you catch weight gain, the easier it is to stop.

You may continue to drift for a pound or two after you make an adjustment to your diet. Don't panic. If you increase your compliance to Drink Your Carbs, using Major Morgan's Grading Scale as your guide, your weight will drift back to your ideal range.

> **Fact:** The best way not to regain lost pounds is to make adjustments the moment you put on three. A side benefit is that you will never be one of those people perpetually whining about how you need to lose five pounds.

Thirteen

What about Gluten and Dairy?

We recently noticed that Frito Lay has been advertising Cheetos as gluten free. We have also seen a proliferation of non-dairy products approximating the color and texture of cheese. Gluten-free and dairy-free foods have become the latest fad in product marketing.

What do we think about this trend? Allow us to answer with a story:

Steven's sister's dog, Max, recently ate a microfiber towel. Even among dogs, Max is known for his iron-clad digestive tract. He has successfully passed pillows, candles and most of a large ottoman. But microfiber proved to be too much for him and the towel had to be surgically removed.

What can we learn from Max? Some things are truly dangerous to eat. Microfiber towels are a perfect example. There are experts who argue that wheat and dairy pose a similar danger. We believe that this threat is a tad overstated.

In his book, *Dangerous Grains,* Dr. James Braley argues that all glutinous grains should be categorized as a poison and stickered with Mr. Yuk.[1] Paleo-diet guru Rob Wolf blames glutinous grains for everything from cancer to schizophrenia and autism.[2]

Dairy has been equally maligned. The far less credentialed authors of the *Skinny Bitch* diet blame dairy products for everything from arthritis and acne to attention deficit and hyperactivity disorder.[3]

We have enormous respect for two out of four of these authors, but we think that they are all unnecessarily alarmist.

Consider the following analogy: it's possible to be attacked and killed by a Chihuahua, but this possibility requires a number of very rare circumstances. Wheat, dairy and other glutinous grains pose a similarly specialized threat. If you suffer from Celiac disease or an anaphylactic response to dairy products, these foods truly are dangerous. For the rest of us, they are not microfiber towels.

Andrea cannot tolerate wheat. Even trace amounts make her sick. Occasionally a restaurant will assure her that a dish is gluten free and then use flour to thicken a sauce. It takes about 20 minutes before Andrea knows with absolute certainty that she has been poisoned. Her symptoms are unmistakable. A rash appears on her chest and cheeks that both itches and gives her the ruddy complexion of an aging alcoholic. Her digestion is wrecked. It takes her the better part of a week to eat once again without stomach cramps and to completely lose that W.C. Fields glow.

Just because wheat is bad for Andrea does not make it toxic for the rest of us. Steven eats very little wheat, but when he does he experiences no negative impact whatsoever. Dairy, on the other hand, is Steven's Kryptonite. It hits him like a low-budget cleanse. Even trace amounts of dairy cause Steven to experience every one of the symptoms listed in the warning labels on Shit Yourself Thin supplements. Andrea, on the other hand, can eat dairy all day with no negative consequences to anything but her calorie count.

Fact: Our two-person sample is enough to illustrate that different people have different dietary limitations. If you don't yet believe us, we have a friend who has no issues with gluten or dairy. Half of a strawberry, however, is more than enough to send him to the emergency room with collapsing airways. Obviously, declaring strawberries hazardous for everyone would be seriously overplaying the threat.

If wheat and dairy aren't poisonous, why does the Drink Your Carbs Food List place most dairy in the "Limited" category and wheat, along with other glutinous grains, under "Avoid?"

We will address wheat and gluten first. In the end, we agree with Dr. James Braley and Rob Wolf. Wheat should be avoided. This is not because we accept their claim that wheat is inherently evil or that it causes autism. Wheat and other glutinous grains simply pack a huge caloric punch while offering few useful nutrients. They don't even do a good job satiating hunger. Go to any restaurant and look around. Most people are capable of eating an entire breadbasket without spoiling their dinner. For reasons we do not entirely understand, people seem able to eat limitless quantities of bread without getting full. This would not be possible with carrot sticks and broccoli.

Dairy is more complex because it has more food value. Dairy can be a good source of protein, dietary fat and minerals such as calcium.

Fact: We recognize that any discussion of the calcium in dairy is controversial and likely to generate hate mail. Experts are mixed on how much of the calcium in dairy is absorbed by the body. It is possible that

> we will eventually conclude that dairy has no more bioavailable calcium than a bottle of Bubble Up. It is equally possible that dairy is being unfairly maligned, much like eggs were a decade ago. Science is awesome like that.

Low-carb diets differ dramatically in their approach to dairy products. The Atkins diet encourages dairy in quantities large enough to drown Sir Milkford the Scholar, cartoon spokesman for the National Dairy Council. Moreover, on Atkins, high-fat dairy is preferable to low-fat and non-fat varieties.

On the opposite end of the spectrum is the low-carb Paleo Diet. The idea behind Paleo is to recreate the diet of our distant, hunt-and-gather ancestors. Since Paleolithic man didn't keep livestock, dairy products are banished from that diet.

> **Fact:** We need to point out that we did not make up Sir Milkford the Scholar. Nor are we now inventing Prince Waffle. If you are a fan of condescending children's literature and poorly drawn cartoons, you can confirm all of this for yourself in the Resources for Schools section of the National Dairy Council website.[4]

We preach a middle ground on the subject of dairy. Our rule is: enjoy non-fat dairy in Unlimited quantities. All other dairy should be Limited.

This recommendation has nothing to do with fat. The reason higher-fat dairy is categorized in our plan as Limited is due to its sky-high calorie count and the fact that, like bread, it's a food that is way too easy to overeat.

Andrea, for example, is capable of polishing off an entire eight ounce wheel of Brie over the course of a single day. On the bright side, doing so would provide her 65 grams of protein. The problem is that all of that delicious protein comes wrapped in 1,500 calories. If Andrea instead consumed non-fat cottage cheese, she would need to choke down pounds of the stuff to reach that same number of calories. She simply could not do it. By sticking to non-fat dairy, you get more food while consuming fewer calories.

> **Fact:** No matter how you slice it, two pieces of bread (wheat or white) total roughly 140 calories. Two square inches of Brie—no one limits themselves to such a small portion, but we will use that number because that is a single serving according to a package we read at the grocery store—is around 200 calories. A couple of pieces of bread and a slice of Brie deliver more calories than half bottle of wine. This is an exchange that no Drink Your Carbs adherent would consider reasonable.

For anyone concerned about the health of Max the dog, he recently ate and successfully passed a rubber spatula. He is doing fine.

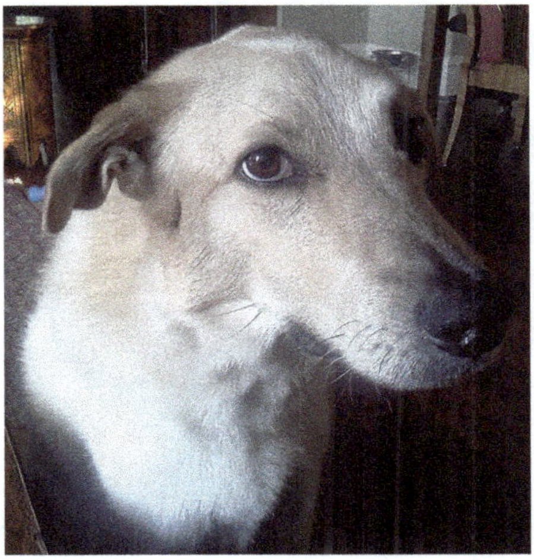

Fourteen

Alcohol and Other Beverages

Every diet has a Boogeyman.

The Atkins Diet Boogeyman is carbohydrates in any form. Consumption of breads and pastas, beans, peas and even fresh fruit are minimized or eliminated because of the carbohydrate count. The same is true with alcohol. All drinking is prohibited during the initial phase of the diet and heavily restricted thereafter. To be fair, Dr. Atkins' animosity towards alcohol was based solely on the carbohydrates. When Dr. Atkins looked at a pint of Guinness Draught, he reeled in horror at the 13.2 net carbs it contained. To put this in perspective, in the Atkin's system a pint of Guinness is the carb equivalent of approximately two-thirds of a pound of foie gras.

To Weight Watchers, large portions are, without a doubt, their Boogeyman. Weight Watchers allows dieters to eat anything they want as long as they don't eat very much of it. The problem is that the typical serving size we have come to expect is two to three times larger than the portion Weight Watchers recommends. As a result, Weight Watchers spends as much time warning members of the danger of eating large portions as Lyndon LaRouche spends warning his followers of the tiny FBI agents hiding in their closets. To Weight Watchers, the whole world is conspiring to over feed you.

South Beach demonizes sugar. They use the term "high-glycemic index foods," but that's just a fancy way of saying their Boogeyman is sugar. Some people get confused because they view starchy foods as different from sweet foods. According to South Beach, they are one and the same. For the record, we agree completely with this basic philosophy. However, South Beach's definition of sugar also includes alcohol. South Beach forbids all drinking in the first two weeks of the diet and greatly restricts drinking thereafter. That's just not for us.

Jenny Craig's Boogeyman is competition. That means any food product not frozen, packaged into cardboard boxes and sold by them directly. The kindest interpretation is that Jenny Craig, by supplying dieters with nearly all of their calories, is able to control dieter's caloric intake and therefore maximize weight loss and ensure the success of the program.

It is equally possible that Ms. Craig is operating in conspiracy with the packaging and microwave industries or that the corporate board simply did the math and realized that selling people every morsel of food that passes their lips is a very profitable business model. Whatever the truth turns out to be, Jenny Craig has made it clear that the Boogeyman is any food that does not bear the corporate logo and cannot be neatly stacked into a tower like children's wooden blocks.

The Drink Your Carbs Boogeyman is Mixers.

Take the Pledge: No More Mixers

When people first hear about Drink Your Carbs, they get excited. The idea that it is possible to lose weight without eliminating alcohol is so revolutionary that it can inspire temporary insanity. This is particularly true when starting out on the diet. We've seen perfectly well-adjusted people happily turn away the breadbasket, swap out the side of potatoes for steamed veggies, and simultaneously undo all that good work by gulping down a 500 calorie banana daiquiri.

Before you kick back and celebrate your new diet with a mudslide or a couple of Margaritas, there is some bad news: as an adherent to Drink Your Carbs, there are some drinks you simply can no longer have. The even worse news is that it's not a small list. Most of the drinks on the "Specialty Drinks" list at your local Applebee's clone are off limits. Toss out most liqueurs, flavored malt beverages and sweet wines. The reason comes back to, once again, calories in versus calories out.

Fact: Not all alcohol is created equal.

- Mixers can turn a 69-calorie shot of Patron Silver tequila into a 400-calorie frozen strawberry margarita.
- Without mixers, the 500-calorie piña colada or 550-calorie mudslide would not be possible. You would have to drink a tumbler filled with rum to come close to those caloric numbers.
- Transforming a glass of red wine into sangria easily doubles the calories with the addition of fruit juice and sweet brandy.
- Adding two tablespoons of simple syrup to your drink increases your calorie intake by roughly the same amount as if you were to dump six packets of white, granulated sugar directly on to your dinner.

Fact: Check our math and you'll find most published calorie totals for the drinks named are half of what we say they are. The reason is that most mixed drink recipes are calculated to a serving size of four to four and a half ounces. Unless you deliberately insult the bartender, you will never be served a drink this small. Most bars serve fruity drinks that average six

> to 12 ounces. Some bars use pint glasses that clock in at 16 ounces. Trader Vic's, a West Coast Tiki Bar made famous by Warren Zevon, serves some of their fruitiest drinks in a "Tiki Bowl" which is the size of a fishbowl and likely contains more calories than a large man should consume in a day.

Pre-bottled, syrupy-sweet cocktail mixers, such as Grenadine, Rosie's Lime and Electric-Green Margarita mix should be avoided as a matter of course. Mixers that advertise themselves as "lower calorie" are no better. Even small amounts of added sugars should be avoided. They might seem insignificant in a single drink, but as a habit, they add up to an enormous calorie load over the course of weeks and months. The addition of just 10 extra calories a day translates to over 3,500 additional calories in a year. According to some experts, 3,500 calories is the magic number that will add a pound to the average person's frame. Whether or not this continues to be true—diet advice from the PhD crowd changes hourly—it is a good idea to avoid adding calories when you just don't have to. It takes some time for your palate to adjust, but you will learn to enjoy unsweetened cocktails or, better yet, your drinks straight up.

Tonic water is less obvious, but equally problematic. A can of tonic water adds about 135 calories to a drink. A can of pre-made Bloody Mary mix rings in at around 80 calories. Both of these choices are superior to a rum and Coke, but neither is a good choice for the drinker who is trying to cut enough calories to lose weight.

As far as we are concerned, sweet wines and sweet liquors are one in the same. The flavor in sweet liquor invariably comes from added sugar. Sometimes sugar is added in the form of fruit juice instead of simple syrup. There are no exceptions for sweeteners—no matter the source. They are similar enough to be effectively the same.

We realize this this categorization is not entirely fair to sweet wines. The sugar in sweet wine occurs naturally. It is the product of incomplete fermentation. Wine makers simply kill off the yeast before the fermentation is complete and the result is a wine with residual sugar. Unfortunately for dessert wines—at least in the Drink Your Carbs plan—this process also leaves them 30 percent to 50 percent higher in calories than a glass of traditional dry red or white wine. More importantly, these wines are sweet; we strongly believe that consuming anything sweet increases sugar cravings. If you insist on an after dinner drink, you are far better off ordering a glass of Pinot Noir, Sauvignon Blanc, or any other dry wine off the dinner menu.

There is a new trend in upscale bars to create specialty drinks that are equal parts unique and pretentious. These new drinks purport to quite literally brim with health. They are organic, natural, locally sourced, filled with anti-oxidants, vitamin enhanced, sustainably harvested, hand-picked, shade-grown, pre-prohibition and fair trade.

Foraged herbs and rare fruits responsibly sourced from remote jungles are used to create flavors that did not exist only six months ago. Perhaps our palates are not refined enough to distinguish the subtleties, but without guidance from the "mixologist" we might never know that we were supposed to taste black pepper, persimmons or bergamot rose. These lists can be tempting. After all, when will you have another opportunity to taste a Martini made with apricot, elderflower and spicy Indonesian curry? As an adherent to Drink Your Carbs, you must learn to resist.

Specialty cocktails are almost always sweetened, even if only slightly, with simple syrup or other juices. It is very rare that one of these drinks will be completely without added sweeteners. The bitterness of the increasingly large menu of things that were never put into drinks but now are, such as wasabi-aged jalapenos, muddled basil and watermelon rind, can only be cut by adding sugar. In our experience, even when sugar is not listed among the ingredients, it somehow sneaks into the final blend. We recently ordered a chili and cucumber martini after being assured that it was completely free of added sweeteners. The resulting drink tasted like Mountain Dew. There is little doubt the mixologist was lying when she insisted that we were "just tasting the natural sweetness of the cucumber."

Specialty drinks are best avoided. The only time you should venture in is if you have a favorite bartender who understands your aversion to mixers and will not lie to you about ingredients, or when your favorite bar adds designated Drink Your Carbs cocktails to the Specialty Bar Menu.

> **Fact:** One of the best things you can do for your waistline is learn to love your coffee black and your alcohol straight up.

Acceptable Alcoholic Beverages on Drink Your Carbs

Wine

- Dry red and white wines are both allowed and encouraged.
- Dry rosé is a good choice as well.

The simple rule for wine is: no residual sugar. Avoid sweet wine. Avoid dessert wine. Wine coolers are similarly forbidden.

> **Fact:** As drinkers, we are as disgusted by wine coolers as vegans are by blood sausage.

This does not mean that wine cannot have fruit flavors. Varietals such as Zinfandel, Viognier and Grenache can be so fruity as to taste sweet without containing any residual sugar. Even the occasional Syrah can seem sweet while technically being dry. The best policy is, if in doubt ask.

- Champagne/sparkling wine is also allowed with one major caveat. Last year, we received a note from a sommelier in Chicago kindly informing us that we knew nothing when it came to bubbly. These wines, it turns out, are often quite high in residual sugar even though they taste very dry. "There is actually only one category of Champagne that contains 0 grams of sugar," she wrote. "It's Ultra Brut, sometimes called Non-Dosage." The best advice we can offer is: if you don't like bone-dry bubbly, keep your consumption limited.

Beer

- Beer is both allowed and encouraged. The only restrictions are that you should avoid sweet beers and try to stick to lower calorie beers overall.

We wish that we could share a few easy rules that would allow you to navigate a beer list and identify the lower calorie options. Unfortunately, as hard as we have tried, we have been unable to correlate brewery, style, color, flavor or even the alcohol content to the number of calories. A 12-ounce pour ranges from around 100 calories to over 300. Fruit-flavored beers are reliably at the high end of the calorie scale. Thicker, sweeter beers, such as Scotch ales and Belgian lambics also tend to pack a lot of calories. Beers designated as "light" are reliably low in calories. The problem is that we have yet to find a light beer with a taste we can tolerate.

Fact: Lance Armstrong claimed to prefer Michelob

> Ultra, but we think the steroids might have been messing with his taste buds.

Until the U.S. Food and Drug Administration decides to mandate nutritional labeling on beer, it will continue to be difficult to identify appropriate beer choices for Drink Your Carbs. For now, the best option we have found is a book by Bob Skilnik, *Does my Butt Look Big in This Beer?* The book lists the calories, carbs and Weight Watcher points for more than 2,000 beers from around the world. Bob spent hundreds of hour sifting through websites and emailing breweries so that we don't have to. It is the perfect resource for the beer lover on Drink Your Carbs. Order it through your local bookstore for about $10.

Hard Liquor

- Hard alcohol consumption is allowed and encouraged.

Avoid sweet liquors, even those that claim to be "naturally sweetened." The best rule is: if it tastes sweet, don't drink it. Clear, distilled beverages are always safe. So is tequila. [Author's Note: By "safe" we mean safe for Drink Your Carbs, not safe in any quantity. Always drink responsibly, no matter what diet you're on.]

Avoid alcohol that has been dyed an unnatural color. We can't think of a single example of a neon blue or fire-engine red liquor that is not sweetened.

Avoid all mixers. We cannot repeat this often enough. Mixers are the Boogeyman. Liqueurs are also out. As far as we are concerned, St. Germain, Hard Tea, etc., are just fancy mixers. Stay away from "diet" mixers as well. Artificial sweeteners are not allowed on Drink Your Carbs.

If you want to add something to your drink, try muddled fruit, pickled vegetables and/or fresh herbs and spices. If you do use muddled fruit, use the whole fruit. Do not accept a pre-sweetened mash. The best methodology for Drink Your Carbs is to crush whole fruit at the bottom of the drink. Spooning mashed fruit from a jar just increases the juice-to-fruit ratio. You can also try floating cut fruit or fresh berries in your drink. Blueberries or strawberries bobbing up and down in a martini glass make your drink downright tropical without blowing your diet.

When drinking a cocktail with fruit, try to make an effort to eat the fruit itself. The goal is not to siphon off the juice. The goal is to eat fresh fruit while enjoying your cocktail.

Fifteen

How Much Can I Drink?

We cannot tell you exactly how much alcohol consumption is healthy. This is not because we believe that alcohol should be limitless. It should not be. The reason that we cannot make a precise recommendation is we have no idea what to recommend.

It would be easy to run with the recommendations from the USDA's Center for Nutrition Policy and Promotion. "If alcohol is consumed, it should be consumed in moderation—up to one drink per day for women and two drinks per day for men."[1] If we thought there was any consensus behind these numbers, we might have adopted them. We are, however, a long a way from agreement between various governmental agencies and researchers.

The International Center for Alcohol Policies maintains a list of International Drinking Guidelines.[2] It turns out that over 30 countries have weighed in on the debate and offered their own recommendations for healthy alcohol consumption. And, as you might have guessed, they differ wildly from one country to the next.

If you accept government guidelines, Italians can safely consume twice as much alcohol per day as Germans and Swedes. Italians can also drink one-third more alcohol per day than the average American. This is according to guidelines published by the Italian Ministry for Agriculture and equivalent agencies in the other countries.

To take these guidelines at face value we would have to assume that Italians are somehow genetically better adapted to drinking. Many of our Italian friends would love to believe this, but we think that conclusion is premature.

Italians are by no means drunken outliers. Spaniards are assured to be healthy while consuming a full 25 percent more alcohol than Italians. In fact, adults hailing from the Basque region of Spain can consume even more. According to the Basque Country Department of Health and Social Security both men and women alike can safely drink a full bottle of wine every single day. We have no idea if anyone follows these recommendations, but it is worth mentioning that the Basque region has one of the highest life expectancies of any region in Europe.

Allow us to share some of the more interesting observations we have teased out of these data:

- You can healthfully drink more alcohol in countries that allow bare breasts to be shown on television. This may be correlation not causation, but we mention it because a possible interpretation is that viewing breasts is somehow protective.
- Austria's government health experts define "hazardous drinking" as beginning at 40 grams of alcohol per day. Coincidentally, this is the same number cited as healthy by Italy, Spain and Japan.
- On the lowest end, the government of the Czech Republic has recommended alcohol consumption at 24 grams of alcohol per day, 15 percent lower than even the puritanical American model. Yet, according to the World Health Organization, the average Czech citizen drinks 74 percent more alcohol per year than the average American.[3] At a minimum, this suggests that the Czech government should consider publishing its recommendations in a larger font.

- Residents of the Eastern European nation of Moldova drink the most alcohol per capita of any nation where consumption is tracked and reported. The committed drinkers of Moldova consume roughly twice as much per year as the average American. Nonetheless, they see no reason to wade into this debate. Moldova has yet to release any guidelines.
- Recommendations for women are typically two thirds of the number of drinks recommended for men, unless you happen to be French, Swiss, Italian, Swedish, Spanish, Basque, Romanian or Australian. Those countries make no distinction for gender. This is either egalitarian or reckless depending on the guidelines from your country of origin.
- On average, members of the Axis powers in WWII may healthfully drink more than members of the Allied forces. We have no idea what to make of this, but felt compelled to point it out.
- The National Institute of Alcohol Abuse and Alcoholism, which is part of the U.S. National Institutes of Health, has put out its own recommendation for healthy drinking. Oddly, their acceptable number of daily drinks is a full 50 percent higher than the figure from the USDA.[4] To be fair, the NIAAA recommendations for weekly consumption are identical to those from the USDA. In other words, if we were to distill the NIAAA position to a T-shirt slogan it would read: "Drink More Less Often."

Consensus is lacking not just between countries, but within them. Last year, the British Physician, Dr. Michael Mosley, stirred controversy on BBC Radio by airing his contempt for the alcohol consumption guidelines of England. When asked for his thoughts Dr. Mosley replied, "Those limits were really plucked out of the air. They were not based on any firm evidence at all."[5]

Although Dr. Mosley was speaking about British recommendations, we are confident that he would feel the same about the guidelines from the U.S. government. First, the U.S. recommendations are nearly identical to those from the U.K. More importantly, Dr. Mosley is convinced that the British recommendations are far too high. If he were in charge he would cap daily alcohol consumption at one-quarter of a pint of beer, or—and we did calculate this—a single shot of Nyquil.

Perhaps Dr. Mosley will be vindicated. Or, in time, it may be deemed healthier to wash down Basque Tapas with a full bottle of vino. We are rooting for the Basque's guidelines, but we will keep an open mind as new studies continue to pour in.

Any recommendation we might offer today would be arbitrary. Our number would be selected randomly from the available sources. We would have no way of knowing if we were right and no way to justify the quantity if questioned. If asked, "How did you come up with that number?" we would be forced to answer with the standard refrain of publishers of creationist textbooks: "Our facts are faith-based."

> **Fact:** We've long been fascinated by the publishers of creationist textbooks. Their decision-making process is so far from our own that we can only imagine the conversations that take place at their board meetings:
>
> "What do we tell people if they ask how we know that Adam and Eve rode a Triceratops?"
>
> "Great question, Jane. First, I'd like point out that this rarely comes up since we stacked the school boards. But if anyone does inquire, show him or her this crudely drawn cartoon depiction. I used it last week in front of a House Subcommittee and they all agreed that it provides more than sufficient evidence."

Before you take our lack of a recommendation as permission to start shot-gunning beers, we want to make it absolutely clear that we think binge drinking is both unhealthy and dangerous. Unfortunately, we cannot say at which drink healthy drinking ends and binge drinking begins. One again, even the vaunted experts disagree.

An often-cited study from the United States sets binge drinking at four drinks per day for women and five drinks for men. By contrast, a study out of Sweden sets the bar at more than twice the American level: half bottle of spirits or two bottles of wine on the same occasion. The Royal College of Physicians in England has entered the fray as well at seven drinks per day for women and 10 for men.[6]

The negative health impacts of binge drinking are universally recognized even if the quantity is still being debated. On the bright side, if you're on Drink Your Carbs you should never hit these limits.

How Much Can I Drink on Drink Your Carbs?

> **Allow us to reiterate a few facts:** We are not doctors. We are not your mom. Nor is either of us a nurse, nutritionist, biologist, anthropologist or anything that might validate our opinion. We have only one advanced degree between us. Steven has a masters' degree in Godzilla.[7]
>
> Ideally this is a question you should ask of your doctor instead of looking for guidance from people who are better qualified to field questions about vintage monster films.

We apply a simple rule to our own lives. Others have successfully adopted our rule as well. It is not a matter of ounces or a number of drinks. Rather, our rule is behavior-based. It is designed to keep alcohol consumption to a reasonable level and provide correction if it gets out of hand. It's so effective that we made it a fundamental part of Drink Your Carbs. Stop following this rule and you are no longer on the diet.

Our answer to 'How much is too much?' is this: Exercise. Alcohol is limited on Drink Your Carbs by the fact that we require exercise. And by "exercise" we mean a serious routine that elevates your heart rate for at least 20 minutes and burns significant calories.

> **Fact:** Exercise should be uncomfortable. That is how you know it is working.

Exercise is not optional. Exercise is required for both overall health and weight loss. Most importantly, exercise turns Drink Your Carbs into self-correcting system. If you can't get out of bed in the morning to fully commit to your workout, you are drinking too much. It's time to dial it way back.

You should never work out with a hangover because you should never drink enough to be hung over. In our own lives, we apply this rule as follows: if a night out partying impacts the next day's workout, we cut our drinking way back. In severe cases, we dial our drinking all the way down to zero, or as we call it, Nightmare Mode.

This rule is probably not sufficient to satisfy the various National Institutes of Health, except perhaps the one in the Basque region. Nonetheless, we have found it incredibly effective. On the rare occasions when we attend a birthday party or wine tasting and drink too much, the feedback is unmistakable. Corrective action kicks in the very next day.

> **Fact:** Instead of a recommended number of drinks or grams of alcohol we offer a biofeedback loop. Or, if you prefer a more philosophical analogy, we offer a Yin-Yang with alcohol on one side and exercise on the other. They must exist in harmony.

One final note to the rare outliers who can drink large quantities and still make it to the gym in the morning: we acknowledge that everyone is different. For most people, our exercise requirement is more than sufficient to cap alcohol consumption at a healthy level. However, there are undoubtedly a few people who can drink right up to the British and Swedish definitions of binge drinking and still function well enough to fulfill the exercise requirement. To these rare few we say: just because you can do it doesn't mean you should.

Ignoring the potential negative health impacts—since you are obviously disregarding them—drinking two bottles of wine or a six pack of beer a day adds more than 1,000 calories to your diet. There is no realistic way to offset a number that large through healthy eating and exercise. Even in Austerity Mode, it would be nearly impossible to offset so many calories. Nor is it realistic to try to burn them in the gym; it would take a nine-mile run. You might be able to do it once or twice—assuming you're not too hung over—but it's just not a realistic daily plan.

In the end, you must find your own formula for balance if our rule is not sufficient. If you find this difficult, you can always fall back on the quantity recommendations of the country in which you reside.

Sixteen

Artificial and Alternative Sweeteners

Some of you are probably asking, "What about diet mixers? Can I have rum and Diet Coke or one of the new sugar-free daiquiri mixes?"

The answer is "No."

We are dead-set against artificial and other non-sugar based sweeteners and not for health reasons. We have no idea which alternative sweeteners are healthier than others. For all we know some of them may be extremely dangerous while others have the power to heal. They may all be bad. They may all be good.

We're not convinced anyone really knows for certain all of the implications of consuming alternative sweeteners. We remember when saccharin was going to save us all from the scourge of obesity. Then one day that all changed; suddenly saccharin became the health equivalent of doing shots of Drano.

> **Fact:** We went to bed one night in a world in which saccharin was a miracle elixir and woke up to find that Tab Cola had sprouted a warning label that read like the back of a tube of model glue. "If ingested unintentionally, induce vomiting immediately . . ."
>
> For more than 30 years, we lived with the knowledge that saccharin is deadly. But it turns out that the last

> word on the subject had yet to be uttered. In December 2010, the EPA removed saccharin from its list of hazardous chemicals. In the EPA's own words, "Saccharin is no longer considered a potential hazard to human health."[1]

Our issue with artificial and other alternative sweeteners has nothing to do with the health effects. Our problem is that these sweeteners taste sweet.

If Drink Your Carbs is followed strictly, your taste buds will adjust to your new diet. After a few weeks of removing most sugars from you diet you will find that your body no longer craves sweet food or drink. It can be difficult at first to avoid a favorite dessert. It is simply a matter of staying motivated and drawing on every ounce of willpower you have. Given a short time, usually a week to 10 days, sugar cravings will diminish.

As they fade, you will learn to enjoy eating healthy foods. This has happened to everyone we know who has decided to dedicate themselves to Drink Your Carbs. Their desire to cheat has gone down while their enjoyment of fresh fruits, vegetables and non-sweetened cocktails has increased exponentially.

Sweeteners interrupt this process. If you eat and drink sweetened foods, even foods without any additional calories, you will continue to crave sugar. The Monkey Brain does not know the difference between real sugars and fake. It's not supposed to. Countless lab rats died in pursuit of chemicals designed specifically to fool it.

The Monkey Brain: Our Most Questionable Scientific Theory

> **Fact:** If proponents of the Paleolithic Diet can ignore evidence that Paleo Man most likely ate more bugs than meat, we too can play fast and loose with evolutionary history.[2]

The Monkey Brain is that part of the human mind left over from our simian ancestors that functions on pure instinct. It is a poo-flinging brute of a creature that has clung to us throughout 65 million years of evolution to wreck havoc on our lives. It is similar to Freud's concept of the Id, except that Freud saw the Id as unconscious while we see the Monkey Brain as very conscious and actively trying to sabotage our plans and intentions.

We have not discussed this theory with an evolutionary biologist. People more qualified than us might deny the Monkey Brain's existence. We nonetheless believe that there is a part of each of us that is still loaded with the original instincts that helped us survive in small bands roaming the savannas of Africa.

It is no surprise that we delight in sweet foods. These foods are calorie packed and, to our distant ancestors, the more calories the better. Imagine if one of our distant ancestors came across a Hostess Sno-Ball dangling like a fruit from a tree. Sno-Balls have so many calories packed into such a small space that, of course, it would taste fantastic. These kinds of dense, easy to obtain calories should taste fantastic to a beast that does not know from where his or her next meal will come.

Unfortunately, the Monkey Brain still believes that every calorie you eat might be your last. As a result, it steers you toward dense calories. The denser, the better. The Monkey Brain implores you to skip the protein salad and instead order a Donut Burger.

If you're not familiar with the donut burger, it's a hit at state fairs across the country. It is a burger with bacon and cheese served with a glazed donut in place of the bun. A donut burger can pack more than 1,000 calories. To the Monkey Brain, it may be the perfect food.

Fact: The people who best understand the power of the Monkey Brain are vendors at state fairs. As proof, we will simply point out that deep-fried Snickers Bars

> have been recently replaced by deep-fried sticks of butter. This is absolutely true. These people are the gods of cheap, fast calories.

Tame your Monkey Brain. If you avoid added sweeteners the Monkey Brain re-calibrates. It will still crave sugar, but it can be retrained to crave the natural sweetness of fresh fruits and vegetables. This may sound ridiculous, but try it before you reject the idea. Avoid all added sweeteners, including those without calories, for two full weeks. Then eat or drink something sickly sweet. We think you will be amazed by the near-instant appearance of sugar cravings.

To this day, if either of us drinks even a sip of diet soda we immediately crave dessert. The Monkey Brain is a powerful force. It cannot be fully defeated, but it can be fooled into craving healthier sweets.

> **Fact:** If Darwin had known that we would spend eight hours a day in front of a screen and drive to any place further than 200 feet from our front door, the obesity epidemic would have been predicted in *On the Origin of Species.*

Seventeen
Sports Drinks

Imagine Coca-Cola running an advertising campaign claiming that the best way to recover from exercise is to drink a can of Coke. The ad is easy to imagine. Kobe Bryant steps off the basketball court to pluck a can from a courtside bucket of ice. He returns to center court and pours a twisting stream of soda into his open mouth. The screen fades to the Coca Cola logo while James Earl Jones reads the voiceover: "For fast recovery, top athletes demand real high-fructose corn syrup." In the parting shot, Bryant hands an unopened can to a kid in the front row who is sipping unhappily on a bottle of water. "Hey kid," Bryant says. "Water's for losers. Winners drink Coke."

The health and nutrition industry would explode into a pick-ax and torch-wielding mob. Advocates for low-carb and low-fat diets alike would march on Coca-Cola's Atlanta headquarters.

A slightly disguised version of this ad runs on a constant rotation on every channel you watch. They are simply promoting a different kind of soda—one without carbonation. The nutritional profile is terrifyingly similar. But because they're labeled "Sports Drink" and dyed day-glow colors instead of brown, few seem to notice or care.

It is true that ounce for ounce, sports drinks contain just over half the calories of a can of Coca Cola. However, sports drinks are typically sold in 24- and 32-ounce bottles. The nutritional labels divide the liquid into smaller portions, but that does little to help. No one in the history of drinking these sickly-sweet concoctions has ever limited him or herself to one quarter of a bottle. Slam a full bottle and you have consumed roughly the same number of calories as Kobe Bryant in our fictional advertisement.

> **Fact:** Sports drinks are Kool-Aid with salt. While brands do vary, you can safely equate a bottle of sports drink to the calories burned in the first mile and half of running. Unless you are running or biking a seriously long distance, sports drinks are not worth it. You are far better off saving those calories for your post-workout beer.

There is a new trend in sports drinks that is certainly healthier than the high-fructose corn syrup based, fruit-free fruit-flavored concoctions. Over the past few years, coconut water has gone from being available only in Thai restaurants to taking over half an isle in our local supermarket.

Bottled coconut water typically contains more calories, ounce for ounce, than traditional sports drinks. Unlike traditional sports drinks, coconut water is sold in smaller containers, thus limiting the damage.

The can we bought for examination was 16-ounces—small by sports drink standards—and dialed in at 120 calories. Drink the entire can and you are within 20 calories of that can of Coca Cola. No matter how we run the numbers, coconut water is not a good choice for people on Drink Your Carbs.

> **Side note to people who believe with a religious fervency that coconut water is healthy because it is packed with vitamins and minerals:** We agree that

> coconut water is a better choice than consuming a combo of high-fructose corn syrup, artificial flavoring and blue dye. This does not, however, make coconut water the best way to get vitamins and minerals into your diet. The best way is to eat fresh fruits and vegetables. Coconut water, by contrast, is not food. It's not in the least bit filling. It adds unnecessary calories without replacing other calories.

There are times when ingesting quick calories in sports drink form makes sense. If you are doing the equivalent of running a half marathon or more you earn enough calories to justify drinking salty Kool-Aid. Otherwise, there are better ways to supplement with electrolytes. Our current favorite is a product called E-Lyte, which is an essentially flavorless concentrate you dump by the capful into your water bottle to create SmartWater at a fraction of the price. There are dozens of similar products. Keep experimenting with them until you find one that works for you.

> **Fact:** So-called energy drinks, such as Monster Energy, often have even more sugar and calories than soda, coupled with a few mysterious uppers that must fall in a FDA/DEA gray area for legality. We mention them here because they are also marketed to sports fans and should also be avoided.

Eighteen

Don't Drive Drunk

A blanket endorsement of taxis, limos, pedicabs, mass transit and all other modes of transportation that do not require us to drive.

As social drinkers, we cannot overstate the importance of letting someone else drive you home. We are so wholeheartedly in favor not driving home that we even extend our endorsement to those unscrupulous cabbies that pick you up at the airport and drive you in circles around the city before finally dropping you at your downtown hotel. If this has never happened to you, it's time to pay a visit to Los Angeles, Las Vegas or New York just for the experience. The reason we include taxicab muggings in our endorsement is that as unscrupulous and maddening as this behavior is, it is still a better choice than putting yourself behind the wheel impaired.

If you are unconvinced by all of the moral and legal arguments you have heard, perhaps we can convince you with a financial one. We have a friend who was pulled over on his way home from a date. He and his date had champagne before dinner, shared a bottle wine during the meal and sipped port for dessert afterward. Dinner cost around $200. The ensuing DUI racked up an additional $10,000 in fines and legal fees. The price is even higher if you factor in the fact that he still pays exorbitant rates for auto insurance based on his newfound liability as a convicted drunk driver.

Our friend is lucky that the damage was financial and emotional. No one got hurt. If he had run into someone . . . well you can imagine how much worse it can get.

He was pulled over for a burned-out headlight. He was arrested. He spent most of a night in jail. He then spent a fortune fighting to keep his license. He spent countless weekends doing his court-ordered community service. On top of all of this, he is still a felon, which he is reminded of every time he fills out a financial form or applies for a job. All of this could have been avoided if he had taken a $10 cab ride, or hell, even $20 if he didn't know the way and the cabbie elected to screw him over.

The math is simple. Let's imagine that you live a long way from your favorite bar or restaurant. Every time you go there, it costs $10 each way. It would take 500 visits to equal the price our friend's DUI. More importantly, during those 500 visits, you can drink with impunity knowing that you are not risking your life or anyone else's.

We chose our current neighborhood largely because of its proximity to our favorite bars and restaurants. When we go out, we typically walk to and from dinner. If we choose a destination on the far side of town, we either take public transportation or call a cab.

Next time you get into a taxi and it smells like body odor and stale cigarettes, just be grateful that you are not behind the wheel. If you happen to get into the rare taxi where the car is clean and the driver is both professional and personable, ask for his or her card. Most drivers will take direct calls. If you are dedicated to drinking your carbs, you should try to keep at least one cab driver on speed dial.

Nineteen

Exercise: A Necessary Evil

Fact: Quick-fix exercise programs and contraptions invariably remind us of the old, Charles Atlas "Dynamic Tension" ads that have been a mainstay of comic books since the 1930s. In just seven days, Atlas claimed, you could pack on visible muscle and learn all of the skill necessary to vanquish a bully from the beach. Sadly, it simply is not true. It was not true during the Great Depression and it still isn't true today. Yet thousands of books, infomercials, magazines and websites still echo Atlas' empty promise. They are all equally untrue, even those that carry the imprimatur of B-list celebrities.

It really would be wonderful if we could spot-reduce fat from targeted parts of the body or make huge strength gains without ever touching a weight. Unfortunately, reality intrudes. Muscle and strength development requires actual exercise. There are no short cuts. It is long past time to banish the Thigh Master to the closet. There is no alternative to getting your butt moving and your heart pumping.

Exercise may be the only thing that diets agree on. Regardless of whether an author recommends that you eat a vegan diet of raw fruits and vegetables or one consisting of zero carbohydrates and as much meat as you can choke down, all require physical activity as part of their program. They may not agree on the type, frequency, duration or intensity of that activity, but they agree on the importance.

Dr. Dean Ornish, in his Program for the Reversal of Heart Disease, recommends moderate walking for 30 minutes per day.[1] On the opposite extreme, some advocates of the Paleo Cave Man Diet endorse exercising at the level of an Olympic champion. Dr. Atkins, in *New Diet Revolution*, splits the difference, recommending moderate walking at first and then intense weight lifting and aerobics as you lose weight and your body becomes more accustomed to physical activity.[2] Even the USDA "MyPlate" requires physical activity. MyPlate recommends 30 minutes, five days a week, and includes a warning that reveals everything you need to know about their target market: "grocery shopping" does not count.[3]

Regardless of the path you choose to lose weight exercise must become part of your life.

If the idea of starting an exercise program causes you anxiety, allow us to offer the following comfort: you are not going to be the most awkward or clumsiest person at the gym. You will not be lifting the lightest weights. Nor, if you join a local road race, will you come in last place. The hideous state of general fitness dictates that no matter how out of shape you feel, you are exceedingly likely to find yourself somewhere near the middle of the bell curve.

And, even if you do come in last place in a race, it is not the worst thing ever. We know this because it happened to Steven. Hopefully his story will offer some calming inspiration.

• • •

[This tale of woe comes solely from Steven. Andrea has never placed last in a road race. She most likely never will.]

I knew I was coming in last the moment we pulled into the parking lot. The race was small. Only 140 runners showed up to circumnavigate the narrow trail around a reservoir in Boulder, Colorado. I could see the other runners gathering near the starting line. The crowd looked far too fit. I didn't know it at the time, but it turned out that a bunch of them were Olympic hopefuls and University of Colorado track stars using the race as a training run. I panicked. I looked around for the weakest person there, and not finding him or her, realized that person must therefore be me.

My original plan was never to tell anyone about my spectacular defeat. I would simply bury it, throw away my race number and pretend it never happened. That might have been an option in the days before race results were posted on the Internet. Google has since made it impossible to hide. Less than two hours after the race I received an email from a friend on the East Coast who runs a ridiculously fast marathon: "Saw the results from the 10k." he wrote. "As far as I'm concerned it's a perfect score: 140 out of 140."

There are other implications of being last. When you are clearly struggling to hold last place people lie to you in the most condescending way. "Almost there!" "Lookin' good." "Lookin' Strong!" They say these things in a tone normally reserved for potty-training toddlers.

Worse yet, by the time I crossed the finish line the food was gone and the beer tent had run dry. One of the many reasons I love Andrea is that she stood at the finish line as I crossed, holding out a beer she'd rescued before the keg tapped out.

I've only come in dead last once. But over the years, I've been passed by every conceivable brand of runner. Old people, young people, people pushing baby carriages and even one guy who weaved his way through a race juggling three brightly colored balls. People have passed me in elaborate costumes, complete with foam rubber heads that clearly make it difficult to breathe. I've been passed by too many children to count, all using the same, sprint-then-walk, sprint–then-walk technique that children seem to favor.

In San Francisco, I once was passed by a hefty, shirtless man wearing tight leather shorts and exquisitely matching three-inch, patent-leather high heels. He made a late move in the last 100 meters of a 5k in Golden Gate Park and I lacked the reserves to stay with him.

Through all of these experiences, I've never once considered giving up racing. And slowly but surely, I have gotten faster. These days I like to tell people, for geeky asthmatic Jewish boys, I'm the fastest one there is. My actual speed is still unimpressive, but within my narrow category I am king.

When I race these days, I'm still passed by runners on both sides like a Toyota Prius trying to keep up on the Autobahn. But no matter where or how I finish, I always finish. In the end, that knowledge gets me back to the starting line.

Twenty

Basic Exercise

If you spend enough time with health and fitness gurus you will eventually hear someone say: walking and running burn the same number of calories per mile. This idea is rooted in eighth-grade physics, or more specifically, the equation "work = force x distance." For those who were distracted or otherwise missed that class, the point is that it takes a defined amount of energy to move a body of mass over a measured distance. The speed of the object is not taken into account. Therefore, running and walking should require the same amount of energy to cover the same distance.

This is usually presented as great news for walkers. "Take a stroll around the block," the thinking goes. "It'll burn just as many calories mile for mile as if you sprinted it." The only problem with this idea is that it's false.

In 2004, four researchers in the Department of Exercise Science at Syracuse University designed an experiment to test the theory. They hooked strangers into a device that measures calorie burn by analyzing breath. We have both been subjected to this peculiar device, although under different circumstances. It involves wearing a facemask connected to small backpack. Andrea likened the experience to running wind sprints in a Darth Vader costume.

Over several days, the test subjects repeatedly ran and walked one mile on both a track and a treadmill. Their calorie burn was measured throughout. The results were astounding. Running not only burns more calories than walking, the difference is enormous. "[T]he cost of locomotion was [approximately] 55 percent lower for males during walking than running, and [approximately] 52 percent lower for females."[1]

In other words, running instead of walking earns you 50 percent more calories over the same distance. This goes a long way toward explaining why all those folks doing slow laps around the inside of a shopping mall don't appear to be losing much weight.

> **Fact:** The authors of this study made another observation that we found equally startling. "There was no difference between the energy expenditure on the track and the treadmill."[2] We have long been told that treadmills are easier to run on because the moving belt does some of the work. Apparently this, like so many other facts we have dutifully memorized, is entirely untrue.
>
> This was not a major conclusion in the study. It was more like a throwaway line in the section describing the data collected. It probably warrants additional research before treadmill manufacturers quote it in advertising. All we know is that if these data hold Steven will never again feel pressure to go running outside in the rain.

Clearly intensity matters. But you don't have to be a runner to take advantage of the metabolic lift intensity provides. A 2012 study from researchers at Colorado State University found that two and a half minutes of all-out effort on an exercise bike can burn as many as 220 calories.[3] For comparison, it would take Steven nearly an hour of slow, casual bike riding to expend that same number of calories.

Drink Your Carb Exercise recommendations are heavily informed by these new data. That said, Basic Exercise is intended for people who do not regularly exercise. It is designed to get folks started and to begin building new, healthy habits. It does demand intensity, but nothing comparable to the cyclists at Colorado State University going all out for two and a half minutes. If you think you are ready for that level of intensity, skip ahead to the Advanced Exercise section.

Walkers

If you're one of those people who absolutely loathes running or biking, by all means walk. This does not, however, mean that you should amble along at the same pace forever. Continually challenge yourself. If you want to burn serious calories, you need to get your heart pumping. There are two ways to do this when walking: increase your pace and/or add an incline. If you live near a hill, walk to the top of it. Increase the pace until you feel uncomfortable. If you work out on a treadmill, use a combination of speed and incline to raise your heart rate. In time, you may even find that you have increased your speed to the point where you are running.

Book Recommendations: The advice we typically offer to people transitioning from walkers to runners is stolen from Jeff Galloway, a man who has written more than a dozen books to coach runners of all levels. Galloway promotes a combination of walking and running. At first, you will find yourself walking a lot and running very little. Over time the ratio will be reversed. You will ultimately be going on long runs punctuated by short walking breaks. In time you may even cut the walk breaks altogether.

We highly recommend Galloway's books. They will have you running far sooner and far faster than any instruction we might offer.

Everyone Else

It does not matter if you are a runner, an elliptical-machine user, stair-climbing enthusiast or user of any of the other cardio equipment found in a typical gym. Our advice remains the same: add intensity and mix it up. Don't use the same machine and don't repeat the same workout every time. Your body will adapt to whatever exercise you throw at it and the benefits decrease. If you always do the exact same workout, your muscles will adapt to that set of particular movements. You'll find that over time you are able to do that workout at a lower heart rate. Your fitness will level out and your calorie burn will actually drop.

Get on a machine you've never used. If you run, throw in an occasional session on a StairMaster. If you typically use an elliptical machine, mix it up with a run on a treadmill. Walkers should take a spin class. Spinners should go for a run. Do something you are not good at. Do something that frightens you. And by "frightens you" we do not mean that you should go out untrained and run a marathon. We mean don't be afraid to look stupid.

Consider taking a Zoomba class or going to an aerobics studio where your incompetence is certain to embarrass you. Embarrassment is good. It means that you are working skills and muscles that have long been neglected. The variation will also help keep you from burning out. Doing the same thing every day becomes soul-crushing drudgery and mixing it up keeps things interesting.

Full disclosure: The extent of our experience with Zoomba is limited to walking past a class and peeking in. We've been making fun of it ever since. They call it a Latin-inspired dance party, but as far as we could tell it was Jazzercise revisited. It was far less cha-cha-cha than it was "Priscilla Queen of the Desert." That said, most of the people in the class looked like they were working hard. So, we say go for it. Just be aware that you are learning jazz hands while being told that you are dancing a Samba.

No matter what exercise path you choose, you must be sure that you're working hard. If your heart rate is not in target zone, you need to do more. Zoomba, aerobics and other cardio classes only work if your pulse is elevated. If the class is easy, you are effectively walking at a slow pace. Based on what we have seen in some classes, it is possible to burn fewer calories than walking. This is absolutely fine, as long as you don't count it towards your daily exercise.

We also recommend throwing some weight-resistance exercises into your routine at least twice a week. We do not, however, recommend that you focus your efforts on weightlifting until you have a strong exercise routine in place.

We have two reasons. First, you can start doing cardio without any kind of plan and with little to no guidance. Pick a cardio exercise and start moving until your heart rate monitor tells you that you are in zone. In 20–30 minutes, you're done. It really is that simple. This is not true of weightlifting.

Without a trainer or experienced partner to show you how to properly lift weights, it is easy to hurt yourself. Lifting with bad form puts pressure on sensitive areas, including your neck and lower back. Unlike cardio, proper weightlifting takes time to learn.

Advice from a doctor friend: "One thing to remember during weightlifting: if it hurts, it's not helping.

> Repeating a lifting exercise that is causing pain might be damaging you. Wearing yourself out on a last set is great. However, lifting through a twinge in your elbow or shoulder might have you wearing an ice bag for a week. Pushing through serious pain may land you in the emergency room."

Equally important, weightlifting will not burn as many calories as a cardio workout. Doing bench presses and bicep curls burns around the same number of calories per hour as a moderate walk on level ground.[4] Upping both the weight and intensity can double the calories burned, but you will still only burn around half of the calories of the equivalent time spent on cardio. While there are numerous health benefits to weightlifting, strength training alone is a lousy weight loss strategy.

Ideally you should do both strength and cardio, but if you have to choose, go with cardio. At the Basic Exercise level, calorie burn is paramount. There will be plenty of time to add strength training as you progress from Basic to Advanced.

Your goal at the Basic Level is to exercise three to four days a week. This translates to a minimum of every other day. The workouts should range from 30 to 45 minutes. At least 20 minutes should be spent in your target heart-rate zone. This will feel uncomfortable. As long as you are not in pain, uncomfortable is good.

> **Fact:** The health and fitness industry is made up of unconscionable liars. They know damn well that their sedentary audience will never hit the gym six days per week. Instead of setting more realistic goals, they lie. They recommend six days of exercise when they're really hoping to get half that many. By contrast, we

> believe that you are grownups who can handle the truth. Three to four days of working out per week is the minimum you need on Drink Your Carbs. If you want to lose weight while continuing to consume alcohol, this is the cost of admission.

Don't panic if you don't have much time to exercise. We understand that life often gets in the way of best intentions. Three to four days a week is a serious commitment. Hopefully you will eventually be able to get there. Until then, don't allow a lack of time to be an excuse to do nothing. If you can only exercise twice a week, by all means do so. If you can only spare 15 to 20 minutes, do a shorter, more intense workout. Starting an exercise program is far more important than how often or for how long you go. You can always add days or duration as your life allows.

If you can only spare 15 to 20 minutes, make it intense. Warm up for two minutes and then push yourself for the remaining time. Remember: the faster you go, the more calories you burn. If you are willing to go hard, you can accomplish amazing things in very short time.

> **Fact:** A short workout should be more uncomfortable than a long one. Think of it as a treadmill colonoscopy: short and difficult but beneficial in the long-term.

If you have been coasting along at Basic feeling like you are capable of doing more, it is time to graduate to Advanced Exercise.

Twenty One

Advanced Exercise

Fact: Beer tastes better when you've earned it. If you stink from the gym so badly that people are fleeing from adjacent tables, this is doubly true.

We have interrogated countless doctors, nurses, athletic trainers and exercise physiologists and they have assured us that you can stick to your Basic Drink Your Carbs workouts and still reap the full health benefits of exercise. There is no need to push yourself to the point that that you end a workout by throwing up. A successful workout is one in which you are within your target heart rate zone for at least 20 minutes. Do this three to four times a week, and you are good to go. When new studies emerge claiming exercise has the power to increase some wellness marker or prevent some hideous disease, you have earned the right to act smug and self-righteous.

That said, if your goal is to be fitter, burn even more calories and/or recapture the vigor of your youth, you'll need to crank it up a notch.

Fair warning: Advanced Exercise requires far more time and effort. Exercise will become a huge part of your life. You will be hitting the pavement or the gym for 45 minutes to an hour, five to six days a week. You will also spend countless hours obsessing, planning, scheduling, agonizing, celebrating and even bragging; it comes with the territory. We all have friends with Facebook pages plastered by their constant athletic achievements. These displays are the adult equivalent of a high school letterman jacket studded with gold-plated pins. Embracing Advanced Exercise will set into motion a process that will very likely lead to you becoming that person. Ignore all of the criticism. As the kid's say, "haters gonna hate."

Advanced Exercise: The Perfect Solution for Your Active, Drinking Lifestyle

Because you will be spending an inordinate amount of time not only exercising but thinking about exercise, it is easy to suffer from burn out. Fitness can begin to feel like work. There will be days when you desperately want to do the equivalent of calling human resources to tell them that you won't be in the office because you've grown weary of your current projects and coworkers. The problem is that, unlike work, exercise is easy to cancel; you simply don't show up. No one calls. No one asks awkward questions. If you miss a workout, only you know. It happens millions of times a day. This explains how your local gym can have 5,000 members yet only one person will be in there working out on an average Thursday morning. To avoid burnout, we recommend focusing your efforts towards a specific sport or fitness goal.

Set a Goal

Your goal can be anything athletic that you find difficult to achieve. A good goal will take a long time and a lot of hard work to accomplish. It should involve gut-wrenching intensity, intimidating duration or, preferably, both. If your goal doesn't fall into either category, you're doing it wrong and you need to choose something more challenging. You will know that you have chosen the right goal when it scares you into showing up for all of your workouts.

> **Note:** Your new, personal athletic goal does not replace your previous exercise program; it's added to your current plan. That is why we call it Advanced.

Goals differ for each person. Common goals include running a marathon, cycling 100 miles or completing a triathlon. However, we know people who have chosen very different objectives.

Our friend David has been laboring for months to swim a full mile in less than 30 minutes. For the record, this is not exceptionally fast swimming. In a triathlon, this pace would place him squarely in the middle of the pack. Michael Phelps could probably swim a 30-minute mile with David chained to his back. But for David, achieving a 30-minute mile will be huge. Goals are intensely personal. What you find difficult someone else might find easy, and the reverse is also often true. For the record, David currently is less than 30 seconds from achieving his goal; by the time you read this, he likely will have succeeded.

A few years ago, Andrea set the goal of being able to do unassisted pull-ups. She set her initial target at five in a row. She could have chosen a running goal, but that would have been playing to her strengths. Andrea is a naturally strong runner. She ran cross-country in high school and college. She has finished marathons. She can run a half marathon at will; in fact, she could probably run a half marathon on no sleep, still drunk from the night before.

When she lacks time to work out, she goes for a quick run around the neighborhood. To Andrea, running is easy. Pull-ups, by contrast, exposed her every weakness. Without some kind of assistance, she couldn't manage a single one.

It took Andrea most of a year to achieve her five pull-ups. Her program involved all of the steps we recommend in Advanced Exercise: five to six days per week of exercise incorporating weightlifting, interval training and mixing up a diverse set of drills and exercises. Andrea did not simply hang from a pull-up bar for 20 minutes a day. That might have worked, but her goal was not to simply develop stronger lats. She wanted to get stronger overall. She wanted to stay physically in balance while progressing towards her objective.

It is possible to ride 100 miles on a bike, do 100 push-ups or a mile of walking lunges without working any muscles not specifically needed for those tasks. We recommend that you resist the urge to focus all of your training on your single-minded purpose. If all of your work is specific to the muscles you will need for a single undertaking, you can throw your body out of balance and make yourself more prone to injury.

Your aim should be to improve your overall fitness. Your goal serves to keep you motivated and allow you to measure your progress. It is a means to an end. The end is a fitter, healthier self.

If You Have Not Done So Already, It Is Time to Add Weight Training to Your Weekly Regimen

The standard refrain encouraging people to start a weight-training program is that muscle burns more calories than fat. The pitch is simple: If you put on muscle mass you will burn more calories throughout your day. That even includes sitting stock-still in front of the television. While the theory is correct, the numbers thrown around are frequently exaggerated. A quick Google search reveals countless fitness-related websites making the same absurd claim: muscle burns, pound for pound, 50 times more calories than fat.

We dearly wish that this were true. Steven converted about 10 pounds of fat to muscle mass over the past two years. He made an effort to lift more and heavier weights and his program worked. If the fitness websites were correct in their calculation, Steven would now be burning 500 additional calories every single day. We assure you this is not the case. Steven's 10 pounds of new muscle mass earn him closer to 60 extra calories per day. Not bad, but nowhere the wild promises made on the Internet.

Fact: "[A] pound of muscle burns six calories a day at rest and a pound of fat burns about two calories a day."[1] These numbers are obviously generalized. Everyone's metabolism is a little different. Nonetheless, it is reasonable to assume that you need to put on roughly 35 pounds of muscle mass to offset one pint of Guinness per day.

To put this in perspective, 35 pounds of added muscle mass would increase Andrea's body mass by over 25 percent. Such gains are possible, but not on the type of program we endorse. It takes a very specific training plan of low repetitions of ultra-high weights combined with dietary changes we would never recommend for non-Mr./Ms. Universe contenders.

If you follow our program you will strengthen and tone your muscles, but if you dream of becoming Lou Ferrigno you need to look elsewhere for guidance.

Muscle unquestionably burns more calories than fat, but we do not think that this should be the primary driver for starting a weight-training program. A far better reason is that weight training is essentially getting a vaccination against sports injuries. A study from the Department of Physical Therapy at Ohio University found that, "resistance training promotes growth and/or increases in the strength of ligaments, tendons, tendon to bone and ligament to bone junction strength, joint cartilage and the connective tissue sheaths within muscle."[2] In other words, weight training strengthens the parts of the body most likely to be injured by the repetitive stress of exercise.

Of course, the act of lifting weights itself carries a risk of injury. British researcher Brian Hamill set out to figure out exactly how big that risk is. He surveyed schools and athletic associations in the United States and Great Britain asking them to report sports injuries. His results were nothing short of astounding. According to Hamill's research, weight training is safer than badminton or squash.[3]

> **Fact:** The sport with the most injuries reported in Hamill's survey was rugby. Steven, for one, was not surprised to learn this. Steven's high school soccer coach—soccer is, according to Hamill, the second most likely sport to injure participants—played competitive rugby with the Denver Barbarians. Since the soccer season ended earlier than most other school sports, the coach thought it would be fun to quickly reorganize the players into a rugby team. He then took the liberty of setting up a few friendly games against other schools that had been playing rugby all season.
>
> The carnage was indescribable. Steven's team never scored a try, or any other points for that matter. It was less of a game than it was a beating. His most vivid memory is of begging to be let off the field.

It is worth noting that Hamill's research was conducted on schools and organized sports clubs. In other words, the data for weight training came from subjects whose activities were supervised by coaches and trainers. Which bring us to the topic of the importance of recruiting an expert for fitness programs.

This is particularly true for weight lifting. Some lifts are highly technical. If you are doing them wrong you are, at best, not getting the full benefit. At worst, you are setting yourself up for months of physical therapy or possibly surgery to correct the ligament you just tore during your one-handed, behind-the-head tricep curl with that 50-pound dumbbell.[4] This does not mean that you have to shell out a ton of cash for a personal trainer. We define expert very broadly. The key is finding someone with extensive experience who is willing to show you the ropes.

Bring In an Expert to Help Guide and Train You Toward Your Goal

No matter how much exercise experience you have, a new physical challenge turns you into a novice. This is a problem that all of us face when setting goals. Figuring out where to start and measuring progress can be difficult.

Andrea worked with a personal trainer to conquer her goal of five consecutive pull-ups. It was expensive, but well worth it. The program completely remade Andrea's body. She lost weight. She gained muscle. She achieved far more than the ability to do five pull-ups.

It's not necessary to hire a personal trainer. Trainers can be outstanding, but there are lower-cost options. We know a guy from South Carolina who decided to run his first half marathon at age 56. He got through it with the help of a $15 book from former Olympian Jeff Galloway. Some people rely on friends who have already accomplished a similar goal to their own and are willing to share their experience. We have lost count of the number of people we know who have been coached through 100-mile bike rides, marathons and triathlons by charity groups like Team in Training and the American Cancer Society. These groups require that you hit up all of your friends and relatives to donate to the underlying charitable cause, but in exchange they will mentor you through the event with coaching, training guides and even group workouts.

> **Fact:** Unless you are attempting to get into the Guinness Book of World Records by doing something no one has done before, it will not be hard to find a website, book, video, friend or professional to help you create your training plan.

Advanced Exercise also demands that you step up the intensity. Increasing the intensity of a Basic Exercise workout is simply a matter of running, biking or swimming a little faster. This is no longer good enough at the Advanced level. It is time to add more structure to your training.

Say Hello to Your New Best Friend: Intervals

For those unfamiliar with the concept, interval training is a methodology that breaks up cardio workouts into periods of near-maximum effort and periods of low effort or even pure recovery. In other words, you might run 400 meters as quickly as you can and then slowly walk the same distance to allow your breathing and heart rate to recover. A standard interval workout might consist of performing this run/walk routine four or five times in a row.

There are thousands of variations of the interval workout, but they all share short duration, high-effort work with defined periods of recovery. These workouts tend to be quicker than a traditional long, slow cardio sessions and they definitely offer outsized benefits for their length. A study from Colorado State University found that people who did interval training not only saw faster improvements in overall fitness, but they continued burning calories at a high rate long after each workout ended. According to the authors, "[study participants] burned an average of an extra 200 calories on the sprint interval workout day."[5]

> **Fact:** Most diet programs begin with the best of intentions. They are founded upon the lofty belief than an idea can make the world a better place. Given time and success, these high ideals are generally abandoned. Diets cease caring about health and fitness and instead concentrate on hawking merchandise. When our day comes, we plan to open a chain of combination interval training gyms and brewpubs with the slogan: "Earn more beer in less time."

Intervals can be done on virtually any piece of cardio equipment. Biking, swimming and running can all allow for an interval workout. We have done interval workouts that involved lifting weights over and over as quickly as possible. Some of our most taxing intervals were performed on a rowing machine. It would be difficult, if not impossible, to design an effective interval workout around a Shake Weight or Thighmaster. Just about everything else is fair game.

Here are a few of our favorite interval workouts. They are short, but do not expect them to be easy. Interval training is hard work. Try mixing them into your program a couple of times a week. We assure you that the additional bump in fitness and calories burned will make the suffering worthwhile.

Classic Intervals: 1, 2, 3, 4 & 5

Some interval workouts require college-level math. Calculating the ratios of work to rest can be maddening. We tend to simplify our intervals because we prefer to focus on exercising rather than trying to calculate two-thirds of 47 seconds.

The goal of this workout is to choose a hard pace you can maintain for all five intervals. We will use running in our example, but feel free to mix it up.

- Run hard for one minute
- Rest for one minute (The goal is to recover as much as possible between intervals. Walk, breathe, stretch, do whatever helps you bring your heart rate down. You may not feel like you need this rest yet. Trust us, you will.)

- Run hard for two minutes (Try to maintain the same pace as you did in your one-minute interval.)
- Rest for two minutes

- Run hard for three minutes (Again, try to keep the same pace.)
- Rest for three minutes

- Run hard for four minutes (Keeping that same pace.)
- Rest for four minutes

- Run hard for five minutes (If you are doing this right, this will be the longest five minutes of your life.)
- Allow your body to fully recover. You are done.

Variation: We occasionally reverse this workout to 5, 4, 3, 2 & 1. It allows us to mix things up. It can also be mentally easier to conquer the five-minute interval first. However, reversing this workout requires some changes to its structure. The goal now becomes going faster or harder in each successive interval. Equally important is to cut the rest time in half. In other words, run hard for five minutes and then rest for two and a half. Run even harder for four minutes and then rest for two. Three minutes of running followed by one and a half minutes of rest. Two minutes of running followed by one minute of rest. One final minute of running and the workout is over.

20 Seconds of Hell: Tabata

Professor Izumi Tabata, an early pioneer of high-intensity interval training, developed a system in the mid-1990s for training the Japanese speed-skating team. On paper it sounds easy: 20 seconds of all out effort followed by 10 seconds of rest. This sequence is repeated eight times. A full Tabata session is only four minutes long.[6] When we were first introduced to Tabata we thought, "How bad can four minutes be?"

> **Fact:** Victims in horror movies invariably fall down while being pursued by the film's monster. Twenty seconds of Tabata will help you understand why. An all out effort is tough to sustain. We do Tabata all the time, yet we have both collapsed to the ground during a Tabata set long before the final eighth round.

The beautiful thing about Professor Tabata's system is that it can be applied to nearly any exercise. Running, rowing, squats, sit-ups and pushups all work. Pretty much any exercise you do can be set to the Tabata tempo.

We often add Tabata sit-ups to the end of a cardio session. We also occasionally design full workouts using the system. We might pick three or four movements such as rowing, body-weight squats and push-ups. We then do each one as a Tabata set. If we are doing three Tabata sets or fewer, we keep moving from one exercise to the next. We sometimes lose a few seconds to the transition, but we like to keep moving when a workout is only eight to 12 minutes long. If we do more than three Tabata sets, we add recovery time in between the sets. We have found that without additional recovery time, our work intervals tend to slow down, defeating the entire purpose of Tabata.

The easiest way to time a Tabata workout is to download a Tabata timer to your smartphone. There are dozens of apps available on every major platform. The timer will chime to indicate that you are supposed to begin 20 seconds all out work. If you are running, you should be at a full sprint. If you are doing push-ups or sit-ups, do as many as possible as quickly as you can. Rest for exactly 10 seconds when the timer chimes again. Do your best to recover as much as possible before the next chime restarts the cycle.

If you follow Professor Tabata's advice and go as fast and as hard as you can during all of the 20-second work intervals, eight rounds will be more than enough time to leave you panting on the floor vulnerable to even the slowest monsters Hollywood has cooked up.

Remember: the key to an effective Tabata workout is to push yourself to your absolute limit during the work intervals. For example, we occasionally do Tabata on a treadmill. We typically do three four-minute sets moving from one into the next without pause. The first set is done with the treadmill set to an incline of 10 or more; we set the speed such that we are barely able to stay on for the full 20 seconds. We then lower the treadmill to half the incline and increase the speed for second set. The final Tabata set is run with zero incline as fast as safely possible. The entire workout takes 12 minutes. Afterward, we feel more wrecked than if we had run five hard miles.

If you are doing a Tabata set of push-ups, squats or other exercises where it is easy to count repetitions, try to hit the same number in each 20-second interval. In the first set 15 to 20 repetitions may not feel particularly difficult. With each successive set, however, hitting that same number becomes seriously challenging. Do not be surprised if you fall short. In the case of Tabata, failure is a sign that you are doing it right.

Adding Intervals to an Existing Workout: Fartlek

> **Fact:** We can be shockingly immature. At times, our inner eighth grader simply gets the best of us and we giggle uncontrollably at things that adults should not find amusing. Fartlek (pronounced "fart-lick") is a perfect example of something infantile that has the power to set us off.

"Fartlek" is Swedish for "Speed Play." At its most basic, Fartlek involves throwing intervals into an otherwise ordinary cardio workout. For example, when heading out the door for a short run, instead of holding a steady pace, add occasional sprints.

Fartlek is as easy to do as it is fun to say. When jogging, warm up for three to four minutes at a steady pace and then choose an object a short distance ahead: a tree, a car, a dog tied up outside of a café, anything. Sprint hard to that object. Then allow yourself to recover for about the same distance keeping an easy pace. Don't worry about perfectly matching the timing of the sprints to timing of the recovery. The point of Fartlek is that it does not have to be heavily structured.

After you have recovered, pick a new object and race toward it. Try to choose objects that will have you running hard for around one to three minutes. The key is to spike your heart rate and then allow it to come back down between intervals. This is easier than it sounds: simply run your sprints hard and then take enough time to recover before you begin again.

The first time you Fartlek, add in no more than a couple of sprints. Over time, work your way up to five or six. Once you have the system down, 25 to 30 total minutes of work is more than enough to earn you a full day of high-speed calorie burning.

> **One Word of Warning:** When you begin your first interval workouts, start slowly. Your first intervals should done be at no more than 75 percent of your maximum effort. You should increase this over time, but it is best to allow your body to get used to the new routine. This will also give you time to learn your capabilities and limitations. For example, if Steven jumped onto a treadmill set to Andrea's top speed he would immediately fly off the back. Starting slowly and learning your capabilities can prevent such misadventures.

Your New Advanced Exercise Plan (A Summary for Skimmers)

1. Pick an extremely challenging and ambitious athletic goal.
2. Find an expert to help you design your training plan. This can range from a high-priced trainer to a low-cost book.
3. Spend five to six days per week training toward your goal.
4. Add weights and other resistance training to your program. (At least twice a week.)
5. Increase your overall intensity through intervals.
6. Diversify your program. Don't do the same workout every time you hit the gym. Mixing it up ensures that you will not over train certain muscles to the detriment of others.

Twenty Two

Insane Exercise

Until now, Drink Your Carbs has been all fun and games. Advanced Exercise is demanding, but it is decidedly amateur. Advanced Exercise is designed to meet tough athletic goals such as finishing marathons and triathlons. The Advanced level of training, however, is unlikely to win you a place on the podium. If your dreams include Olympic gold, or even just taking your athletic endeavors to the highest level possible, you will ultimately find yourself flirting with Insane Exercise.

> **Fact:** Insane Exercise exists because some people don't know when to stop. This is not a bad thing. If some people were not born without a pause button, we would have no Williams sisters, LeBron James or Laird Hamilton.

Anyone looking for a detailed Insane Exercise plan is going to be disappointed. Insane Exercise is incredibly personal and extremely sport specific. No one would train a swimmer using a fitness plan designed for a sumo wrestler. No NFL lineman could expect to maintain his muscle mass on a weightlifting plan designed for a professional cyclist. The training plan a friend used to prepare for the CrossFit Games was completely different from the plan our podiatrist used to train for the Western States

100-mile Endurance Run. Training is always sport specific, but at the Insane level it becomes laser focused.

If you want to elevate your game to the highest level, you will need the expertise of a coach or trainer. We are unqualified to fill this role. We periodically try to step-up our exercise to the Insane level. Every time we attempt it—with its required six days a week of exercise, obligatory two-a-days, higher weights and even greater intensity—we end up battered, exhausted and in more or less terrible shape. Neither of us has yet to sustain this level of exertion for longer than two weeks before a strain, pulled muscle or, in one case, a blister straight out of a medical journal that engorged Andrea's big toe into an overripe plum forces us to dial back. This is the great unknown of Insane Exercise. Some people can hack it and some—ourselves included—cannot. The only way to find out is to try. Trust us when we say that your body will let you know into which category you fall.

> **Fact:** Andrea's blister was bad, but it was nothing compared to a show-stopping injury suffered by an old friend. That friend popped his bicep deadlifting north of 400 pounds. At the top of the lift, a tendon snapped and his muscle rolled up like a window shade. The friend is fine, by the way; he had the tendon reattached and he's as good as new. Steven, on the other hand, is still haunted by the sound.

If your body can withstand the effort, Insane is the path to your athletic best. The rest of us will have to be satisfied at the Advanced Exercise level. It's nothing to be ashamed of; you can spend your life working out at the Advanced level and be among the fittest people you know.

The question that must be answered is, if Insane Exercise

is intended for people who train at the elite level why is it even included in Drink Your Carbs?

We have all been told a certain fairytale that elite athletes are teetotalers. The myth is that these athletes match their brutal exercise regimens to an equally regimented diet. They approach food as nutrition and balance their protein, carbohydrates and fats to whatever mystical ratio is the current fad among Jamaican sprinters. They avoid unnecessary calories, especially the empty ones in alcohol.

There are, most certainly, athletes who adhere to highly restrictive, booze-free diets. We have actually met a few of them, although they have been few and far between. We have met a far larger number of professional athletes—and people who workout as hard as professional athletes—who live a lifestyle far closer to Drink Your Carbs. They may not call it Drink Your Carbs. At times it may not even look like Drink Your Carbs. They do, however, follow the basic model of eating a super-healthy diet and rewarding themselves with alcohol. They work out crazy hard. Eat crazy lean. And they drink, often as hard as they exercise.

Years ago, we witnessed most of the starting lineup of the Denver Nuggets basketball team stumbling into a bar with their entourage. It was during the NBA season, but obviously not on a game night. They proceeded to consume more beer than we would have thought humanly possible. We did not count their drinks because we did not want to stare. Even if we had stared, it unlikely we could have compiled an accurate figure. It was too many, too fast. All we can say is that if either of us drank that many pints we would have left that bar in the back of an ambulance or police cruiser.

We have a friend who competed in the 1984 Olympics and describes the scene at the Olympic Village as a booze-soaked bacchanal. To hear her tell it, most of the athletes kept to the straight and narrow until they were done competing. The moment medals were awarded in their particular sport they unleashed their inner Keith Richards. Apparently, Olympic athletes are bound by the same secrecy rules as members of the Cosa Nostra. She refuses to share the kinds of details and scandals that sell books. But she will divulge that the competitors in the 1984 games behaved exactly as you might expect from an unsupervised group of over 7,000 young, sexy, super-fit 20-somethings. A few athletes returned home with fame, glory and medals around their necks; everyone else returned home with a wicked hangover and crab lice.

We know plenty of athletes who were, while playing for their college teams, locked into hotel rooms on the night before big games because their coaches knew that without supervision they could not be trusted. For the record, that lack of trust was completely warranted. Studies have shown that college athletes binge drink more often than their non-athletic peers.

We have more than just anecdotes to prove it. Researchers at Harvard University's School of Public Health surveyed more than 12,000 students at 130 colleges and universities and found: "Among male subjects, 57 percent of athletes reported at least one binge drinking episode in the previous 2 [weeks] compared with 48.8 percent of non-athletes. Among female subjects, athletes also reported a higher rate of recent binge drinking (48 percent) than non-athletes (40.2 percent)."[1]

The correlation between athletics and heavy drinking does not end at college graduation. A New Zealand study on the subject found "frequent binge drinking was reported by elite provincial level sportspeople (58 percent), closely followed by elite international/country level sportspeople (54 percent), non-elite (44 percent) and non-sportspeople (35 percent)."[2]

Clearly, there is more drinking among top athletes than is covered by ESPN. This is the reason that Insane Exercise exists. We strongly believe that many of these athletes could benefit from a more measured approach to alcohol. Moreover, current scientific research supports the assertion that moderate drinking—even if that drinking is done more frequently—is far more compatible with athletic training.

So far, we have ignored the physiological effects of alcohol on exercise and post-exercise recovery. Alcohol makes little difference to the amateur athlete, provided you stick to the amount we recommend. If, however, you are trying to squeeze every ounce of performance out your body, there are a few alcohol and exercise related factors you should take into account.

There is no shortage of opinions on the effects of alcohol on exercise, but surprisingly few studies have been done on the subject. This may be because it is a difficult subject to study. Alcohol tolerance and athletic performance are both highly variable and dependent on difficult-to-control factors such as fatigue, hydration and diet. Setting up a well structured, reproducible experiment is no easy task. There is the additional hurdle of getting approval from a university's clinical research ethics committee to study the effects of an intoxicating substance on human subjects.

> **Researchers:** "If you would please skip to page 14 of the proposal. Under the heading "Non-Random Controlled Experimental Design" you will see that our plan is to get people drunk and set them loose on a basketball court."
>
> **Ethics Committee:** "Rejected. That said, if you find another university to sponsor the experiment we want tickets to the game."

The study most often cited by those who claim alcohol and exercise are incompatible was published in 2010 by a team of researchers at Massey University in New Zealand.[3] It was a small study involving only 11 participants. All of the participants were men. This is far from ideal; it is too small and too lacking in diversity to be used for broad claims. Nonetheless, the experiment, which was designed to test the direct effect of alcohol on muscle recovery, is genuinely clever.

Each of the study participants was placed—sober—on a seated leg extension machine. The participants then performed 300 single leg extensions while an attached computer took detailed notes on the length, strength and speed of their repetitions. Three hundred repetitions of any exercise is more than enough to work a muscle to complete exhaustion. All of the participants reported major soreness the following day. Although the study fails to mention it, it is very likely that many of those participants awoke so sore that they had difficulty lowering themselves onto the toilet.

Fact: Nearly everyone who has played around in a gym has likely used some form of the machine used in the study. You are seated so that your knee bends over a cylindrical pad and your shin locks in behind a weighted lever. Straightening your leg against the resistance isolates and flexes the quadriceps muscle.

Outside of rehabilitation centers, the seated leg extension is losing popularity. Most of the bodybuilders and trainers we know have quit using it altogether. They insist that the machine puts unnecessary strain on the knees and you can get the same results with less risk by doing weighted squats.

After each participant completed his exercise, he was fed either a glass of orange juice or a screwdriver cocktail. In theory, the juice drinkers were the control group, but we have a hard time believing that they could not tell if their drink contained alcohol. The cocktail recipe was a ratio of 3.2 to one, orange juice to vodka. This is far from a stiff drink, but it was more than sufficient to identify the vodka in our unscientific taste tests.

The total amount of alcohol administered to each participant—excluding the control group who drank pure juice—was equal to one gram of alcohol for every kilogram of body weight. The alcohol was consumed within 90 minutes of completing the exercise. Unfortunately, the study does not detail participants' resulting blood alcohol content. But the authors do note that "the volume of alcohol consumed . . . is enough to be considered as binge drinking."[4]

Fact: In order for Steven to consume one gram of alcohol for every kilogram of body weight, he would need to drink a six-pack of beer or a little over one-third of a bottle of vodka. As important as the quantity is the speed of the intake. The liver is an impressive organ, but 90 minutes is a very short time to process that much alcohol.

We considered replicating the drinking portion of the experiment. Fortunately, more sensible heads prevailed and we instead consulted a chart published by Brown University. Assuming the chart is still accurate for people beyond college age, Steven's blood alcohol content would be approximately .12 percent. The chart further details the anticipated effects of such blood alcohol level. "Coordination and balance becoming

> difficult; distinct impairment of mental faculties and judgment."[5]
>
> This undoubtedly explains why the study's authors felt compelled to mention: "Once the required amount of beverage was consumed participants were driven home and instructed to go directly to bed."[6]

Over the following three days, the participants returned to the lab to do additional leg extensions. All of the participants saw a drop in their strength after doing the initial 300 repetitions. Muscles take time to recover after exercise, so an initial drop in strength was expected. The drinkers, however, lost more strength. The greatest difference was observed on the second day. The non-drinkers had lost 19 percent of their leg previous strength. The drinkers had lost 34 percent. On the bright side, it appears that the drinking delayed recovery rather than terminated it. By the third day following the exercise, both the drinkers and non-drinkers were regaining their strength at similar rates. The authors' concluded: "alcohol magnifies the severity of skeletal muscle injury and therefore delays recovery of strength . . . participants in sports containing intense eccentric muscular work should be encouraged to avoid alcohol intake in the post-event period if optimal recovery is required."[7]

From this reading, you'd think alcohol and athletics couldn't safely mix. Muscle recovery is required for strength building and no athlete wants his or her recovery affected or delayed.

Fortunately, for those of us who enjoy both drinking and exercising, the story is far more complicated.

A year after the study was first published, the same group of researchers repeated their experiment, but this time they cut the amount of alcohol in half. Over 90 minutes post exercise, the participants were served one-half gram of alcohol for every kilogram they weighed. In Steven's case, this would amount to three beers or just over half a bottle of wine.

With the alcohol dose lowered, the results were strikingly different. The follow-up study concluded that the "consumption of a low dose of alcohol after damaging exercise appears to have no effect on the loss of force associated with strenuous eccentric exercise."[8]

What have we learned? Alcohol can delay muscle recovery after exercise, but it appears to be highly dose dependent. We hope the researchers in New Zealand continue testing different alcohol levels. In the mean time, if we want more granularity on how much alcohol one can drink before affecting exercise recovery, we have to look at an earlier study done by a team at the University of Massachusetts. The alcohol dosage used in that study fell between the other two, .8 grams of alcohol for every kilogram of body weight.

There were a few key differences in the UMass study. All 10 test subjects were women. Instead of using leg extensions, they used bicep curls. Blood was taken every day for five days after the exercise to track markers of muscle recovery rather than testing directly for loss of strength. And most importantly, they administered the alcohol before the exercise. In other words, they got a bunch of ladies tipsy and dragged them into the gym.

> **Fact:** The cocktail administered in the U. Mass study was quite a bit stronger than the cocktail in New Zealand. "The alcohol used was vodka (80 proof) which was mixed with equal parts of orange juice and cranberry drink."[9] We have no idea what this cocktail is called, but it is only a splash of peach schnapps short of Sex on the Beach.

Ten days after the initial study, the test subjects were invited back to do the same bicep curls with their opposite arm. This time they were not dosed with alcohol in advance. When researchers compared results from the two sets of blood tests, they found no significant differences.[10]

> **Fact:** Assuming there is little difference between drinking right before exercising and drinking right after, Steven is now at five beers or nearly a full bottle of wine without affecting his post-exercise recovery.

Of all of the studies of alcohol and exercise we have seen, the one that interests us the most has yet to be published. In late 2011, Dr. Manuel Castillo of the University of Granada School of Medicine presented preliminary findings to the 11th Annual European Conference on Nutrition. His PowerPoint presentation, which is available online, was entitled, "BEER AFTER EXERCISE: Yes or No?" Considering that drunken tourists account for the lion's share of Grenada's economy, it is not surprising that Dr. Castillo's answer was a resounding "yes."

Dr. Castillo had 16 men run on a treadmill for 60 minutes in a room heated to 95-degrees. It was the cardio equivalent to Bikram yoga. The goal was, quite simply, to make the men sweat buckets. Dr. Castillo then allowed the men to rehydrate by drinking as much water as they pleased. Two weeks later, the men repeated the treadmill test, but this time each man was given 22 ounces of beer followed by as much water as he pleased.

> **Fact:** A 22-ounce bottle of beer is referred to as a "bomber." It is roughly equivalent to two beers, assuming one foams over a bit onto the table.
>
> Dr. Castillo did not serve his beer from a bomber.

> Included in his presentation are photographs of a sweaty, shirtless hunk of a man drinking lager from a large graduated cylinder.

If you have ever watched one dog inspecting another at a dog park, you understand the level of scrutiny Dr. Castillo applied to his study participants. After both of the treadmill/hydration tests, each man was given a full checkup and put through a DEXA x-ray body composition scan. Blood, saliva and urine were collected. Vision and reflexes were tested. The participants were even subjected to a multiple-choice exam. Dr. Castillo did everything short of requiring a semen sample.

Dr. Castillo did not test his samples for markers of muscle recovery. He instead looked for indicators of rehydration. He wanted to know if alcohol after exercise dehydrates the drinker. His results made headlines around the world. The body scans, blood, urine, saliva and test scores all concurred. Subjects were more hydrated after drinking beer and water than when drinking water alone.

> **Fact:** The final slide of Dr. Castillo's presentation sums up both his and our enthusiasm for his research. Beneath a montage of a pouring beer and a man leaping into the air in the classic victory pose were the words: "RUN! ENJOY! BE HAPPY!!!"[11]

Here is what we think know about alcohol and exercise, using Steven as our example: The alcohol equivalent of six beers in the hour and a half after exercising will delay Steven's muscle recovery by about 36 hours. Three beers over the same amount of time will have zero effect on Steven's recovery. The equivalent of five beers consumed in only a half an hour also appears to have no effect on recovery; we are less confident about this one since the study subjects consumed their alcohol prior to exercising which is something Steven refuses to do.

If Steven wants to ensure that alcohol will not negatively impact his exercise recovery while taking advantage of its hydrating effects, the magic formula appears to be two drinks. Two drinks is well below the threshold affecting muscle recovery while offering the benefits of improved hydration and higher scores on some multiple-choice exams.

> **Fact:** The multiple-choice exam administered by Dr. Castillo was designed using the Vienna Test System. There is no need to look this up on the web; just picture the monitor from an Apple II+ attached to the button console from the classic arcade game Defender. Unfortunately, we have to wait until the study is published to learn exactly what questions were asked.
>
> For now, we will simply accept Dr. Castillo's results as confirming that a couple of beers also improves the play of videogames from the pre-Dragon's Lair era.

Additional and more comprehensive studies will be helpful. For example, we would like to see different types of alcohol tested separately. We currently accept the U.S. Centers for Disease Control assertion that "[i]t is the amount of alcohol consumed that affects a person most, not the type of alcoholic drink."[12] However, it may turn out that wine, beer and hard liquor have different physiological effects when it comes to exercise recovery. We hope that the teams in New Zealand and at UMass will consider rerunning their experiments using beer or wine instead of vodka cocktails. We similarly hope that Dr. Castillo's shirtless beer drinker will show up in a future presentation sipping on a glass of shiraz.

Nonetheless, the presently available studies are more than enough to convince us that drinking alcohol is fully compatible with serious athletics as long as athletes are not binge drinking. In other words, the current drinking pattern of many competitive athletes is exactly the wrong approach.

For anyone who still doubts the need for Drink Your Carbs among elite athletes, we want to share a final case study. We considered writing about our friend Trent who competed in the CrossFit Games. We considered interviewing our friend Willie who played in the NFL. Trent did not drink while he was in training. By contrast, in his NFL days Willie drank like pregnant women eat. In the end, we decided that either story would be too traditional for Drink Your Carbs and better suited to the pages of *Sports Illustrated*. We elected instead to step outside the box and feature Chip the Chippendale.

Case Study: Chip the Chippendale

"Chip" is not his real name. Since he is now the CEO of a large fitness company, we promised to conceal his identity. He was not a competitive athlete in the traditional sense. He was a Chippendale dancer. His exercise regimen was every bit as rigorous as that of any professional athlete in the world. He truly fits the definition of Insane Exercise.

Chip assured us that his diet and exercise program was not unique among the dancers. Apparently, they all used similar schemes to keep their trademark Chippendale washboard abs. The Chippendale workweek consisted of two shows on Friday and Saturday nights. Since the dancers brought home between $1,000 and $1,500 a night, most of them did not bother to hold a day job.

They instead spent their time working out, tanning, waxing and otherwise getting ready for the next weekend's performances.

Chip worked out twice a day between Monday and Friday. He did intense cardio in the morning. He lifted heavy weights in the afternoon. Five two-a-days a week is the very definition of Insane Exercise. Chip also ate close to no carbs. From Monday to Friday, his diet looked like the Atkins Induction Phase, except that he also limited his fat intake because limiting fats further restricted his calories. Chip ate no sugar. No fruit. No starches, including rice, wheat, potatoes or even high-protein grains like quinoa. He drank no booze. It is also worth mentioning that over the course of the week Chip also restricted his water intake in order to slowly dehydrate himself; apparently dehydration is a key component of the chiseled look of Chippendales' abs.

> **Fact:** That Chip was able to cope with the dehydration and stay healthy when most of his calories came in the form of protein powder is a testament to the resiliency of the human body.

The moment the curtain went down on the final show on Saturday night, Chip morphed into Caligula. Starting at three in the morning, just after the end of his shift, Chip began an unrestrained cheat day. For 24 hours, he ate and drank anything and everything he desired. He typically began with cocktails at an after-hours club, followed by a breakfast of a dozen donuts. By noon, he was washing away the previous night's hangover with mixed drinks and piles of fried appetizers. Lunch and dinner were one continuous food orgy. It was one mountain of simple carbs after another, with little break in between. Chip's only rule was that the party ended Sunday at midnight.

> **In defense of our Caligula analogy:** We have it on excellent authority that there is nothing disparaging we can say about Chip's after-hours behavior during his Chippendales days that doesn't fall short of his actual conduct. Also, since we are not using his real name, he is unlikely to sue.

There is no denying the fact that Chip's diet worked. His body fat hovered around 6 percent. His abs stayed stripper-perfect. He was able to exercise at an unbelievably high level. He was always ready for his weekend performances.

Why then do we think that Chip would have been better off on Drink Your Carbs?

The minute Chip stopped dancing, he ballooned by 60 pounds. In less than two years, he went from the fittest guy he knew to showing signs of metabolic syndrome. The Chippendale diet worked for the same reason that all diets work: the calories Chip took in each week balanced with the calories he burned. It didn't matter that he took in most of his calories on Sunday. He burned those extra calories doing two-a-day sessions in the gym. The minute he stopped dancing, however, he reduced his workouts and relaxed his diet during the week. His caloric intake quickly outstripped his calories expended.

We know that Chip's calories balanced while he was dancing because he maintained a perfect 6 percent body fat. We also know that on his cheat day, Chip drank easily seven days worth of alcohol and ate up to 5,000 empty calories.

Drink Your Carbs did not exist when Chip was dancing. If it had, we strongly believe that it would have allowed Chip to maintain his pay-him-to-take-his-clothes-off physique without the trauma of binging and starving. Drink Your Carbs would have given Chip the structure to keep his carbohydrates and calories low. By staying in Austerity Mode and scattering his drinks throughout the week, his overall calories would have remained constant. Instead of his Sunday food orgies, he would have lived a far more pleasant life throughout the rest of the week.

Most importantly, Chip might have developed eating and drinking habits that could be maintained after he retired from the stage.

• • •

If, after hearing all of this, you still want to give Insane Exercise a try, here is our best advice. Get a coach. Create a plan. Say "goodbye" to your spouse, friends, significant other and/or children because you will rarely see them. Assuming your body can take the abuse, all of your free time will be spent training.

Of course, since we are unable to maintain Insane Exercise for any length of time, our insights are modestly worthless. We will leave you instead with some simple, straightforward advice from our friend and coach Trent. As Andrea was stepping onto the floor to compete in a small, local CrossFit competition, he puffed his chest, clapped his hands and said: "Get out there and fucking crush it."

Twenty Three

Incorporating Exercise into Your Life

Andrea has exercised for virtually her entire life. Steven, though starting a little later, has exercised regularly for more than 20 years. We have both been professionally coached. We have regularly sought the help of experts in our quest to become healthier, fitter and leaner.

Unfortunately, this does not make us personal trainers, nor does it qualify us to dispense advice on how others can best integrate exercise into their own lives. In other words, the fact you have had an appendectomy does not qualify you to perform one. Lucky for us, we are friends with a man who has over 50 years of experience training athletes. He was kind enough to share his hard-earned wisdom.

Willie Hector was drafted to the NFL's Los Angeles Rams in 1961. His selection for the team is even more impressive in the context of the time. In the early 1960s, the NFL had unspoken quotas; there was no written rule, but it well understood by everyone involved, from the owners and coaches to players and staff, that teams would limit the number of African-American players. The L.A. Rams were one of the NFL's most integrated teams in 1961 with a full 25 percent of positions on the roster filled by African-American athletes. The Washington Redskins, by contrast, remained an all-white team until 1962 when they integrated only in response to Kennedy Administration threats to evict them from their publicly owned stadium. In other words, at the time Willie entered the NFL, he was part of a large population of black athletes competing for a very limited number of positions on each roster.

> **Fact:** A bit of history of race and professional football: The early 1960s represents the only era in which the Canadian Football League was competitive with the National Football League in play quality. The reason, according to most historians, was that the CFL was far more integrated. A lot of African-Americans who were locked out of the NFL by quotas went up to Canada to play ball. In fact, after being cut from the Rams, Willie played a few years in Calgary before returning to the United States for a partial season with the Denver Broncos.

Willie always knew that the career of a NFL lineman was likely to be short. A few players are able to stick around for a decade, but most last no more than four or five years before injuries retire them. During his time off between seasons, Willie earned a Master's Degree in Physical Education. When he left the Broncos, he hung up his jersey, walked out of the locker room and never looked back. He retired this year after half a century of teaching and coaching at both the high school and college levels.

> **Willie Hector Fact:** Willie's Master's thesis was titled "The Effects Of Foods on An Athlete's Performance

Prior to An Athletic Contest." His conclusions, by modern standards, seem mundane. When Willie was playing professional football, standard nutritional advice was to eat as much protein as possible in the 24 hours before a game. The pre-game meal endorsed by the NFL in his day was a buffet spread featuring the entire hindquarter of a cow. Staff and trainers were on hand to encourage the players to eat as much as possible. Since no one wanted to eat right before a game, these meals usually took place the night before. Nonetheless, Willie has strong memories of getting to the field still feeling like he'd consumed a lead brick.

Willie's thesis put forward the radical supposition that a pre-game meal balancing complex carbohydrates with varied protein sources was easier to digest and would therefore improve performance. The typical reaction these days is, "duh." At the time it was far more controversial. There were more than a few old-school professors who viewed that thesis like Pope Urban VIII viewed Galileo's heliocentric model of the universe. If they could've thrown Willie in front of the Inquisition, they most certainly would've done so.

We cannot overstate Willie's influence in our lives. We've known him for nearly 20 years. We still call him first when we have questions about exercise, fitness, injuries, diet or any thing else performance related. We are obviously not alone. Almost everyone we know calls him "Coach."

Fact: Watching a football game with Coach is one of life's great pleasures. Coach obviously knows the game

> very well, so his commentary is far better than anything said on television. But the real fun comes when the camera pans the sideline. Coach still knows a ton of people in the NFL, especially among the coaches and coordinators who are closer to being his peers. And unlike TV commentators, Coach isn't bound by a code of secrecy. Coach's color commentary usually includes the unpublished back-story to hirings and firings. Sometimes, he'll even share the salacious details behind a high-profile divorce.

The first time we called on Coach's expertise was shortly after we met him. Steven had just begun learning the basics of Olympic Lifting. He found that holding a barbell in front of him in "rack position" was wrecking havoc on his wrists. Steven has a tendency to panic at the first sign of pain or discomfort. He was convinced that he had permanent nerve damage.

> "If you lay off for a day or two, does it get better?" Coach asked after listening to Steven whine.
>
> "Absolutely," Steven answered. "But the minute I start lifting the pain starts again."
>
> Coach relaxed visibly. "Take it easy for a few days. You'll be fine."
>
> "This doesn't feel fine."
>
> "As long as an injury gets better when you take time off, you're fine," Coach said. "It's the injuries that don't get better that you have to worry about."
>
> We still quote this advice all the time.

When we have questions we always go back to Coach. He has forgotten more about health and fitness than we will ever know.

Exercise Advice from Coach Willie Hector

Define Your Goals

Coach often points out that most professional athletes retire well before their 40th birthday. There are a few outliers such as swimmer Dara Torres and Hall of Fame wide receiver Jerry Rice. But most professional athletes stop competing well before then. "They don't stop because they want to," Coach explains. "They stop because they have to."

The ability to bounce back from injury is a rarely mentioned factor that makes a huge difference in the longevity of athletic careers.

Competing professionally puts a lot of stress on the body. These athletes are working themselves to the edge of their capabilities. As a result, they occasionally get injured. The question then becomes, how quickly and completely do they recover from those injuries?

Coach doesn't bring up the possibility—or even likelihood—of injury to discourage people from competing. Quite the opposite. If you want to compete, Coach will cheer you on. He mentions the potential of injury solely because it's a major factor to be considered when defining your fitness goals.

For example, if your goal is not to beat the Williams sisters on the tennis court but rather to still be playing club tennis in your 70s and 80s, your daily workouts need not resemble the daily drills undertaken by the Williams sisters. Working out like the Williams sisters can increase your risk of injury. Backing off, by even a little, allows you to stay fit and healthy while reducing the injury risk.

This is why Coach recommends defining your fitness goals up front. If you want to compete at an elite level, you should push as hard as you can and see if your body can take it.

If your fitness goals fall short of world domination, Coach argues that pushing yourself to the absolute limit is not required. That said, Coach is still a strong advocate for competing. You'll maintain a higher level of fitness if you participate in competitions, even the casual road race or tennis round robin. He just sees a big difference between training to complete and training to win.

Listen to Your Body

Coach is adamant that everyone should exercise regardless of age or fitness level. However, throughout his long career, Coach never tried to produce a one-size-fits-all exercise program.

"Everybody is different," Coach says. "It's impossible to standardize for people with different goals, different abilities and different levels of fitness." The one piece of advice he offers to everyone he has worked with is, "Listen to your body."

"I don't care if your muscles hurt," he told us. "In a day or two, you'll be fine. But if your joints or tendons ache you need to pay attention."

His reasoning is simple: joints and tendons recover slower than large muscles. If you don't give them time to heal when they've been overstressed, a slight ache can progress into a chronic problem.

Let your body be your guide and listen to its cues. If you start feeling pain in your joints, tendons or vertebrae, back off and take it easy for a few days.

But, Coach warns, "Don't use minor pain as an excuse to stop exercising," Instead, go light or change up the type of exercise you're doing. If you run, try biking. If you bike, try swimming laps. The goal is to maintain your exercise program while letting your tendons and joints recover.

Coach's Tips

Set Your Patterns Early

"People who are not active when they're young are rarely active when they get old." Once eating and exercising habits are set, they are far more difficult to change. This does not mean that you are doomed if did not work out in your 20s and 30s. But, the sooner you get into healthy patterns, the easier they will be to maintain.

Start Today

No matter how old you are, you can find the right exercise program. It will inevitably have to change as you age, but scaling back is a much better option than cutting out exercise altogether.

We'll use Coach as our example of how exercise programs can change and adapt as we move through our lives:

In his 20s and 30s, Coach ran up to three times a day. He would run once on his own and twice with the track teams he was coaching. He lifted heavy weights three times a week. One of his favorite exercises during his NFL days was to push his car around a parking lot. You might have once had to push a car across the street to a gas station; Coach is the only person we've ever met who actually enjoyed it.

In his 40s and 50s, Coach started biking and walking. He began to scale back his weight lifting. He lifted regularly, but he lowered his weights to around 75 percent of his maximum capability. He also took more time off between workouts. This is, according to Coach, one of the keys to healthy aging. Your recovery time slows as you age. "Once again," he say, "pay attention to your body and give yourself time to recover between workouts."

Now that he's in his 70s, Coach walks. Most mornings he reads his newspaper while trudging slowly up an imaginary hill on his treadmill. He still lifts weights, but he now holds himself to 55 percent to 65 percent of his max. He is no longer trying to add to his fitness. He is now simply fighting to maintain. He expects to be fighting this fight into his 90s and beyond.

Fuel Your Body

We have not mentioned this yet, but Coach has been living an approximation of the Drink Your Carbs Lifestyle since the late 1950s. He eats healthy foods, he exercises and rarely does a day go by when he fails to pull the cork on a bottle of wine or pour himself an evening glass of Jack Daniels.

One of our favorite ways to eat in San Francisco—a city with some of the best food on the planet—is having dinner at Coach's house. It invariably includes a big salad, his famous BBQ chicken thighs and/or ribs and enough wine to kill the Roman God Bacchus.

Long before First Lady Michelle Obama began her anti-obesity campaign, Coach was advising his students on the importance of eating well. "Think of your body like a car," he likes to say. "It you put bad fuel in it, it's not going to run well."

Most of his advice comes down to: avoid sugar and processed foods, and be sure to eat plenty of lean meats, fresh fruits and vegetables.

Like all of us, he has had to reduce his calorie intake as he has aged. These days he favors a low-carb approach. More than once we have watched him push away a breadbasket or a basket of corn chips and say, "I'm saving these calories for my wine." In the end, this may be a better summary of Drink Your Carbs than any description we've come up with so far.

We wish everyone had Coach in their lives, and hope many of you have your own version. If not, we are happy to have shared a few insights from one of the smartest and wisest men we know.

Twenty Four

Travel

At home, adhering to Drink Your Carbs is easier. You control your purchases at the grocery and liquor stores. When you eat at home there is no excuse for not eating healthy foods and drinking mixer-free drinks. On the road, however, all diets become more difficult. Travel often means being faced with a series of poor choices.

> **Fact:** In some cities, even the salad comes breaded and deep-fried.

Strange bars in unfamiliar towns tempt you with impossibly cheap drink specials mixed in primary colors and served in tall, seductive glassware. These are drinks specially designed to appeal to the same parts of the brain that attract magpies to bright, shiny objects. Sometimes those evil bastards even let you keep the glass as a souvenir, bringing together the deadly combination of eye-catching dyes, our addiction to sugar and our general fondness for anything free.

On the road, temptations are everywhere. This is entirely by design. Wherever you are in the world you can be assured that the local Chamber of Commerce has conspired with the City Council and local businesses to find ways to fill your belly and empty your wallet. They have full-time employees whose job it is to be the tiny devil standing on your shoulder whispering bad ideas. If their seduction fails, they simply do more market research until they find some newer, more compelling combination.

> **Fact:** Somewhere in the world there is a team of food scientists trying to figure out how to serve a piña colada in a glass made out of a funnel cake.

In order to prove that Drink Your Carbs is the perfect solution for a weight-gain free, guilt-free vacation, we embarked on five Drink Your Carb trips to very different locations around the world. We took the Drink Your Carbs diet to Las Vegas for a three-day weekend. We visited New York to see how Drink Your Carbs stood up to some of the greatest restaurants in the world. We traveled to Antarctica to test Drink Your Carbs in one of the harshest environments on Earth. We ate and drank our way through the Middle East. And, finally, we journeyed to the island of Crete where we discovered the most perfect Drink Your Carbs food ever conceived.

Twenty Five

Travel Case Study: Las Vegas, Nevada

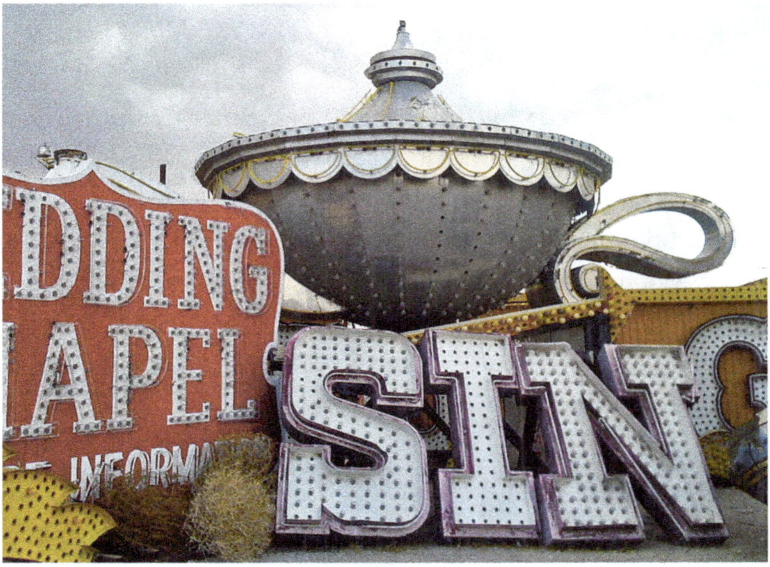

The moment you touch down at McCarran International Airport, your senses are overwhelmed by the sights, sounds and smells of Las Vegas. The sights and sounds are provided by the rows of slot machines incessantly flashing and dinging in the terminal.

Question: How big of a gambling problem do you have if you can't even wait until you get to your hotel?

The smells are courtesy of fast food, of simple carbs and grease. When hungry, these are some of the most compelling smells in the world. They promise cheap, fast, easy calories. No matter how well we eat, no matter how dedicated we are to our diet, we freely admit that these smells still give us the classic Pavlovian drool response. And Las Vegas' McCarran Airport ups the stench factor higher than anywhere else we have ever been. Some of these smells were so powerful that we wondered if the cooking fans were vented directly into the terminal. It is for times like this that we try to live by the following:

Rule: Never land hungry.

"Never land hungry" is the first rule of Drink Your Carbs travel. It was also the first rule we violated. We worked out the morning before our flight and somehow miscalculated how much time it would take to get back home, finish packing and leave for the airport. We made the flight with plenty of time to spare, but we had to skip lunch in order to do so. Ideally, we would have filled one of our carry-on bags with healthy snacks. But this too was thrown aside in the rush.

Eating food provided by the airline was out of the question. The calories in in-flight meals come almost entirely from simple carbohydrates. We have long maintained that if you are going to break the rules at least break them for something worthwhile. The best in-flight meals fail to meet even the low standards of a high school cafeteria. It is as though the airlines deliberately tasked a team of food scientists to create a Hungry Man Dinner knockoff with twice the calories and half the pleasure.

We were ravenous when we landed.

Neither of us is good at being hungry. Andrea's patience vanishes. Her patience for things slow or incompetent is never particularly high, but when she is hungry she has no tolerance at all. As her blood sugar drops, she transforms from her mild-mannered self to Mike Tyson trying to bite your ear off.

Steven is no better. If not fed, he tends to throw temper tantrums like a two-year-old in the cereal aisle. His head drops. His shoulders slump. His walk slows to a reluctant shuffle. In short, when Steven is hungry he becomes everything that makes a hungry Andrea explode.

After years of marriage we have learned to manage these situations by recognizing them and steering ourselves toward food. Only one of the two of us typically recognizes the situation. The other is too deeply in the grip of a hypoglycemic fit. This may be one of the great arguments in favor of partnering for life. When one of you is stuck in an irrational pit of hunger-induced despair, the other person usually stays rational enough to search for food. Furthermore, it is our experience that even if food isn't present, as long as we know we will eat at some point relatively soon, we can temper the worse of our behaviors.

As we landed in Vegas, Andrea took charge.

"We are not stopping in the airport," she said. "Keep moving and I promise we'll eat before we get to the hotel."

Steven's moping slowed us only a little as we cut across Vegas toward our first Drink Your Carbs meal at In-n-Out Burger.

Fact: When traveling, food is a series of compromises.

We are not fans of fast food. The quality is as low as the calories are high. Next time you are in a fast-food restaurant, look at how much of the kitchen space is dedicated to fryers. This should tell you everything you need to know. While it is true that McDonald's and Burger King have added salads to their menu, boxed salads get about two square feet of shelf space while a full third of the kitchen is dedicated to cranking out fried food.

The only conclusion to draw is that McDonald's and Burger

King keep a few salads on display behind the counter as window dressing, to give the impression that they care about your health. Clearly no one orders them and they add no revenue to the bottom line. We wouldn't be surprised if they are eventually replaced with the same kind of plastic food that is on display in the windows of Japanese noodle shops.

> **Fact:** Wendy's Baja Salad clocks in at 740 calories, 47 grams of fat and 1,990 milligrams of sodium. This would be a travesty if anyone had ever ordered one.

In defense of fast food, it is, true to its description, fast and readily available. For this reason, we all occasionally find ourselves eating it. The key to the Drink Your Carbs lifestyle is finding ways to eat at these restaurants without completely blowing your diet. There is no excuse for hitting Carl's Junior and gorging on 2,000 calories of French fries and artificial-strawberry milkshakes. Super sizing your meal might seem prudent because the additional 1,200 calories cost only pennies more, but find a way to resist. The goal of any trip into a fast food chain is to eat just enough to sustain yourself until you can find decent food later, and to do so without blowing all of the calories you are planning to drink later that night.

The way we manage fast food is to walk in with the full intent of sticking to Drink Your Carbs. As we crack the door and the smell of grease wafts out, we have been known to repeat the words, "We are going to drink our carbs," over and over like the chant at the end of a yoga class. This does not mean that we are planning to order beer with lunch. We mean that no matter what delicious bargains are offered on the Dollar Menu, we are sticking to the rules of Drink Your Carbs. In this case, our grand entrance sounded more like:

Steven: "I don't care anymore. I don't even want a burger."

Andrea: "Stop it. You're just hungry."

Steven: "I'm not hungry. I'm fine."

Andrea: "Just shut up, I'm ordering you a double hamburger, protein style."

Steven: "Whatever."

Most fast-food restaurants have options that work with Drink Your Carbs. In-N-Out Burger makes it particularly easy. Any burger can be ordered "protein style," which replaces the bun with large pieces of iceberg lettuce. It's a burger salad served in the style of an ice-cream sandwich. Is cold lettuce really a satisfying replacement for a toasted bun? No, but skipping the bun is not that great a loss. More importantly, skipping the bun saved us 150 calories each, which we knew we would need later when we hit our first casino bar.

We matched our "protein style" burgers with plain iced tea. We skipped the fries. It was a small meal by any measure, but it served its purpose. It gave us the lift needed to check into our hotel, unpack our bags and head downstairs for a mid-afternoon snack at the tapas bar in the City Center Casino.

City Center looks like Superman's Fortress of Solitude as envisioned by an eight-year-old with an Erector Set. While the design came from a fancy architect and cost just shy of $10 billion to build, the exterior looks unfinished. The interior is more coherent, assuming that it was intentionally built to mimic a hamster Habitrail.

Fact: The greatest architectural minds in the world

have conspired to ensure that once you are inside a hotel casino you cannot find your way back out. A side effect of this type of design is that it is equally impossible to find your way through a casino or to find anything inside a casino. This is just fine with the architects as long as it keeps you lost among the slot machines.

The Spanish tapas bar, Julian Serrano, is located in the front of City Center, so it took us nearly 20 minutes to find.

Andrea: "I think we've been through here already."

Steven: "I don't think so."

Andrea: "I recognize that old lady.

Steven: "You're sure?"

Andrea: "Watch her for a second. She'll take a drink from her daiquiri without taking the cigarette out of her mouth. She kind of swings it to the side."

Steven: "Fair enough. Your turn to lead."

Julian Serrano is a restaurant scaled to its surroundings. The space is huge and dark. The ceilings are cavernous. The tables seem to go on forever. Large, exterior windows do nothing to brighten the space. The restaurant somehow maintains a late-night ambiance even in the early afternoon.

Fact: The American Institute of Architects has done itself a huge disservice not granting Julian Serrano an award for Masterful Use of Window Tint.

The menu was just as difficult as we had hoped. We chose tapas because they pose a significant dietary challenge. We could have gone for sushi; as long as you focus on sashimi and avoid tempura, sushi is one of the easiest foods to eat on Drink Your Carbs. We decided instead to begin the trip by testing our will power. Spanish food is difficult on Drink Your Carbs because carbs are staples of the diet. Rice, potatoes and bread are ubiquitous. The menu at Julian Serrano was no exception. The *paella*, which is a Spanish name for a giant pile of rice with saffron and mixed seafood, looked incredible. As did the *patatas bravas*, which is comprised of fried potatoes smothered in spicy mayonnaise.

We ordered a bottle of wine as soon as our waiter greeted us. "You really should consider the sangria," he replied.

Steven took the lead. "We're in Vegas for a Drink Your Carbs weekend. Mixers are strictly forbidden."

"There are no mixers in our Sangria."

All sangria is some combination of wine, fruit juice, some variety of sweet liquor or brandy and frequently, simple syrup. His personal definition of "mixer" must have been as limited as ours is broad. "We appreciate the offer," Steven replied, "but we'll stick with the white. Also, please do not bring any bread. We don't need it."

> **Rule:** Never let the server bring bread to your table. Letting a breadbasket sit on your table is the equivalent of a recovering heroin addict allowing a friend to store morphine in his refrigerator.

We stuck largely to meat and vegetables. This is not to say we were perfect or that we successfully avoided all simple carbs. Again, when traveling, food is a series of compromises. The chorizo turned out to be paired with small, boiled potatoes, but instead of rejecting the dish, we simply left most of them behind. The shrimp bubbling in garlic and olive oil presented a bit of a quandary in that it could very much be considered deep-fried, given that the shrimp was about waist high in oil, but we ordered it anyway after confirming that is was not breaded. It is worth remembering that most diners who order similar dishes sop up every drop of oil with baguettes. Simply avoiding the bread and the excess sauce can easily eliminate 500 calories with minimal impact on a dining experience. These are the types of compromises that make Drink Your Carbs work.

Fact: If you need motivation to stay on your diet in Las Vegas, just look around.

We were immediately reminded of why we are so strict with our diets the moment we found our way back through the casino and out onto the Strip. It was late afternoon. The lights of the hotels were in full bloom. The sidewalks were jam-packed with human traffic meandering at an impossibly slow pace. Nearly everyone on the street was obese. It was even more shocking to see how many of these people had, hanging from nylon cords around their necks, huge souvenir glasses filled with brightly colored daiquiris.

We tried to figure out how many calories are in a daiquiri served from a repurposed Slurpee machine into a four-foot plastic replica of the Eiffel Tower. Our best estimate is well over half of the calories any reasonable person should consume in a single day.

Rule: A drink that comes with a souvenir cup is automatically disqualified from Drink Your Carbs.

Vegas-Specific Rule: If you want to avoid the crowds just take the stairs.

We ducked into the Bellagio for a quick drink, both to get away from the crowds and to take a moment to digest some of what we saw on the Strip. There was one man in particular who stood out to both of us. He was so large that he was having difficulty walking. His knees no longer bent under his weight, so he moved by swinging his legs around side of him as though he were on painter's stilts. Around his neck hung a souvenir glass from the Hard Rock Café molded into the shape of a plastic guitar. The glass was almost as big as a full-size Fender Stratocaster. It was filled with thick blue liquid. When the man was not sucking on his cigarette, he slurped the blue liquid through a two-foot straw.

Andrea ordered a glass of rosé wine. Steven ordered a pint of Guinness. The rosé had been opened for too long. It tasted a little like the refrigerator it was stored in. The Guinness was fine. We did not see it poured, but from its lack of thickness Steven guessed that it came from a can. We toasted to another round of mixer-free drinks, and wondered aloud if that man on the street was intentionally trying to kill himself. He was unquestionably in the process of committing suicide. The only question was whether he was doing it on purpose.

"It's got to be intentional," Steven said. "Look at it this way. Imagine being that guy's doctor. He comes to you and says, 'I'm trying to commit suicide in a socially acceptable way and I need some ideas for how I can speed the process up, how I can kill myself faster.' I don't think I could help him. Every suggestion I could offer, he's already doing. He smokes. He clearly doesn't exercise. We've seen his taste in booze. I can't imagine his diet gets better from there. It has to be deliberate because he is being so thorough. If he asked me 'Is there anything I could do to speed up my death?' I'd have nothing for him. I'd tell him to keep up the good work."

We cancelled our reservation at some fancy Italian place at the Wynn and instead opted for sashimi at a nearby sushi bar. Sometimes, you just need a role model to convince yourself that you're on the right path.

Still a little hazy from all of the wine and saké, we dragged our butts down to the gym the next morning and did an hour of speed work on the treadmill. We wouldn't normally work out quite that hard on vacation, but we knew that later that night would be our big, blow-out meal. We needed to feel that we earned the right to eat it.

> **Rule:** For every big meal you have on vacation, do one intense workout in the hotel gym. This effectively limits the number of big meals you eat because no one wants to spend their holiday doing two-a-days.

The other reason that we decided to run hard was that if we had not been able to complete a tough workout, we would've had to cut back on our drinking. Since neither of us wanted to face this possibility in Vegas, we faked a smile and ran hard. Only afterward did either of us admit how difficult that run had been.

> [**Editor's Note:** Seriously? These two are the Johnny Knoxville of health and fitness. No way Legal is going to rubber stamp a recommendation that people workout hung over. We'll be sued by some idiot who flies off the back of a treadmill still drunk from the night before. At a minimum we need one of those drug-ad disclaimers: "Ask your doctor: 'Is working out hung over right for me?'"]

There is a certain feeling of triumph that comes from walking into a restaurant still dripping sweat and stinking from the gym. This is doubly true in Las Vegas. As we stepped into the hotel café for breakfast after the workout, we could see panic spread across the hostess' face. Her eyes darted back and forth from our sweat-soaked t-shirts to her seating chart. She was obviously doing spatial geometry in her head, trying to figure out which table would place us the absolute furthest from ruining other diners' experiences. It was an impossible task in a full restaurant. She finally settled on a small table near the back, sandwiching us between an older man in a Sean Jean sweatsuit that had clearly never seen sweat and a young couple still dressed for evening cocktails. Neither party looked particularly pleased to see us.

When eating out, we tend to spy on what other people are eating and drinking. Sean Jean sweatsuit was not a small guy and he was working his way through a huge stack of pancakes topped with a scoop of butter the size of a baseball. The couple on the other side, clearly reaching the end of a long night on the town, were both quite trim. The man was well dressed in jeans and a fitted gray t-shirt. The woman wore a classic little black dress cut well above mid-thigh. They were sharing the remainder of an egg white omelet and nursing the last of a bottle of champagne. Clearly they were adherents to Drink Your Carbs, even if they didn't know it yet. We were so impressed that we mimicked their order, except for the champagne. We drank black coffee in deference to the fact that, while they were ending their day, we were starting ours.

We considered spending the day in a casino underneath the haze of secondhand smoke. We rejected the idea when we looked outside our hotel window and realized that the sun was shining without a cloud in the sky. We grabbed books and headed downstairs to find a shady patch alongside the pool.

It has been argued that it's a mistake to think that just because you worked out in the morning, that you've earned the right to sit around doing nothing for the rest of the day. It's based on the idea that you undo the benefits of the exercise by spending fewer calories then you would have on a typical day. We respectfully disagree. As long as we work out in the morning—and avoid all the mixed drinks and deep-fried goodness on the menu from the poolside bar—we are perfectly happy to lounge. The difference between the calories we would have spent in a casino and the calories we did spend poolside is too minimal to concern us. So we spent our day relaxing. We barely had to move. They brought a lunch of burger salads right to our cabana.

That night was the meal for which we had been saving up our calories. We promised ourselves one big dinner where we would not obsess over every morsel. Picking the restaurant was not easy. Some of the greatest restaurants and renowned chefs from around the world have opened Las Vegas outposts. We considered a multi-course French blowout with the seal of approval of the Michelin Tire Company. We considered any one of the seemingly endless versions of high-end steak joints, but steak and broccoli is one of our standby meals so it did not feel special enough. We even considered a classic Vegas buffet, but we dismissed that idea as very likely to be not worth the calories.

We finally settled on a Thai restaurant in an off-the-strip strip mall dominated on one end by an enormous Swingers Club. We might have missed the Swingers Club, but our taxi driver took great delight in pointing it out. Our driver was clearly a fan of the place. He was shockingly specific about the décor and services offered. He kept repeating the fact that there was a couples-only area, as though this would be the selling point that would pique our interest. For the record, had we been swingers, the couples-only area would have been a complete turn off. It is safe to assume, based solely on the existence of a restricted couples-only area, that the rest of the club must be overrun with creepy single men.

"Take a brief respite from the constant, unnerving harassment," seems to us to be a weak slogan for attracting couples; perhaps as a single man our driver missed that implication. He also seemed particularly impressed by the fact that the club had a spa where communal hot tubs bubble away like egg drop soup.

By the time we got out of the cab in front of Lotus of Siam, we both needed to wash our hands.

Lotus of Siam is both a complete dive and—as of this writing—probably the best Thai restaurant in America. The location feels vaguely unsafe. The parking lot is a little too dark. The bars on the windows of the adjacent liquor store are a little too thick. If not for the constant flow of people coming in and out of the restaurant, the place would feel downright dangerous.

> **Fact:** Someone once sent us an article from some long-forgotten British Journal that claimed eating spicy food triggers weight loss. The argument put forward was that consuming capsicum, the ingredient that makes peppers hot, creates a metabolic boost and for hours afterward your body burns more calories than it otherwise would have. Lotus of Siam is clearly cooking for adherents to the theory. We played it safe, ordered our food medium-spicy, and wound up what was probably the spiciest food we have ever eaten. The garlic shrimp appetizer was habanero hot and garlicky enough that we both still reeked two days later. At times it was difficult to continue eating, but the flavors were so good that we could not stop.
>
> We are not adherents to the "spicy foods = weight loss" theory. Our reason has nothing to do with the

> science behind the study, which we have been unable to locate. Our reason for rejecting the connection is that if it were true, Frito Lay would be advertising that fact to promote Flamin' Hot Cheetos.
>
> Let's face it: all the big snack-food companies, including Frito Lay, Hostess and Sara Lee, have armies of scientists who are paid to find and verify these exact kinds of claims. Think of the branding potential. The moment these companies decide the results of this study are solid enough to be defended in a lawsuit, the market will be inundated with Spicy Twinkies and Sara Lee Five-Alarm Cinnamon Rolls. Until this happens, we can all safely assume the connection between spice and weight loss is far from confirmed.

We broke nearly every rule of Drink Your Carbs that night. No fried foods: we started with egg rolls. No simple starches: we ladled two different curries onto beds of perfectly fluffy, white rice. No added sweeteners: we finished the meal with mangoes and sticky rice, which is made from slices of fresh-cut mango resting on a bed of sweetened rice, drenched in a sauce that is probably half palm sugar. It was a diet buster all around, which means that the meal went according to plan.

As we mentioned, there are times when all of us fall off our diets. Sometimes these lapses are intentional, sometimes not. The key is to get right back on the very next meal. A lapse isn't a failure unless you decide to make it one. We woke up the next morning and hit the gym for a quick weight session before a solid Drink Your Carbs breakfast of eggs and fresh fruit.

We both returned home from the trip without gaining a single ounce.

Andrea, in fact, came home a pound lighter than when she left. This was somewhat unexpected. Our goal was not to lose weight. By drinking our carbs, we were simply trying to limit the consequences of eating and drinking to excess, which naturally happens whenever we go on vacation. The goal going into any trip of this sort should be to limit the damage. You don't want to come home five pounds heavier. An added pound or two can usually be shed with a few days in Austerity Mode. Any more weight gain than that and it takes serious work to undo the damage.

We did better than expected in Las Vegas, and we did so without feeling like we gave anything up. That's the power of Drink Your Carbs.

Fact: "What Happens in Vegas Stays in Vegas" can be applied to unwanted weight gain.

Twenty Six

Travel Case Study: New York, New York

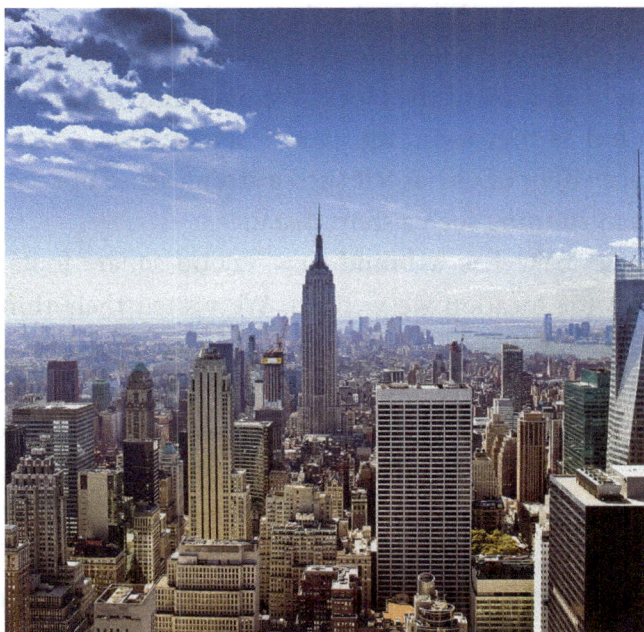

There are few feelings worse than the mix of horror and disgust you get when something drips on you from above while you're walking down a sidewalk in New York. It may be just condensation from a window mounted air conditioner. We always assume these drips are either an experimental virus carelessly spilled from an unlicensed medical laboratory or some hideous comic-book style mutagen. It's bad enough that no one in New York cleans up after their dog, leaving the entire city littered with landmines. Some days, navigating the three blocks from our Chelsea apartment to the subway was like walking from South Korea into North Korea through the DMZ. The minute we focused our attention on the ground, the assault began from above.

On top of the landmines and random dribbles, the sidewalks are piled thick with trash bags, scaffolding, deliverymen pushing dollies with boxes piled high, tourists scanning maps and people in suits shouting obscenities into cellular phones. All these obstacles came together on the day we dropped in on CrossFit Black Box NYC for a noon workout. The warm-up included an 800-meter run around the block. We now fully understand how salmon feel as they swim up river to spawn. It has been a long time since either of us has felt such a strong sense of accomplishment from running such a short distance.

CrossFit NYC has a brand new 12,000-square-foot facility. That's not the location we went to. We visited their third floor location in the Flatiron District. The space would've made a perfect live/work loft. It had high ceilings and great light streaming in through large windows. As a gym, however, a three-story walk-up is difficult because you can't drop weights without risking the lives of the people in the suite below. As far as we could tell, they manage this by not doing a lot of Olympic lifting at this location. This restriction, however, didn't stop them from kicking our asses. Our workout included handstand push-ups, pull-ups and burpees. Andrea finished in the middle of the pack. Steven came in dead last.

Fact: The coaches at CrossFit NYC were awesome. The members were helpful and incredibly welcoming. The only thing that could've made our experience better was if they'd had a balcony. A perfect end to the workout would've been to step onto a balcony to catch our breath and cool down. And we could've become a part of New York's eerie landscape by dripping sweat onto unsuspecting strangers below.

Running around the block was not the only time we risked our lives for a good story for this book. At the hyper-expensive, mind-blowingly delicious, West Village Japanese restaurant, Nara, we ordered a course of tempura-fried blowfish. Battered and fried food is definitely not on Drink Your Carbs, but we ordered it anyway just to see if blowfish would kill us.

Fact: Prepared incorrectly, blowfish is deadly. Blowfish contains a powerful neurotoxin, tetrodotoxin, which shuts down communication between nerves. There is no known treatment or antidote. Cooking the fish does nothing to reduce the toxicity. Symptoms begin with difficulty speaking as the central nervous system is slowly paralyzed. Over the next few hours, the lungs and heart stop receiving instructions and quietly shut down. It's better than having your face eaten off by zombies, but slow suffocation is most certainly an unpleasant death.

Prepared properly, blowfish is as safe as any other fish we eat. In reality, the risk is tiny. No one has died of blowfish poisoning in years. But a chance of death, no matter how small, adds a layer of drama that most other foods lack. You get to pretend you're playing Russian roulette while doing something less risky than eating oysters.[1] (We love oysters. We eat them all the time. Nonetheless, this is absolutely true.)

For those not interested in sampling blowfish for themselves, we'll describe it. Blowfish is tasty. It's a light flaky white fish. If we'd been told it was cod, we would've said it was the best piece of cod we've ever tasted. Our lips didn't tingle. Nor did we experience hallucinations. Our speech remained clear, at least through the first bottle and a half of sake. In spite of the fact that blowfish commands street-drug pricing, it turns out that it has none of the side effects.

The final risk we took in pursuit of a noteworthy vacation was to shun hotels and instead book an apartment through the website Airbnb. If you're not familiar with Airbnb, it has the power to turn every single person in America into an innkeeper. Have a moldy tent in your garage? Set it up in the back yard and, with the help of Airbnb, you're now the proprietor of the worst bed and breakfast in America. They also list whole houses and apartments. Since we're too old and grouchy to go back to having roommates, we opted for an empty apartment in Chelsea.

> **Fact:** Renting an apartment is by far the easiest way to travel on DYC. If you have a kitchen, you can shop and cook. Being able to fully control even one meal a day makes a huge difference in limiting your dietary damage. At a minimum, it's nice to be able to make your own breakfast, which is always the most difficult Drink Your Carbs meal to eat out.
>
> It is usually possible to order a Drink Your Carbs-friendly omelet and a side of fruit, but most breakfast menus read like a dessert course. Avoiding sugar and simple carbs at lunch can be challenging. Avoiding sugar and simple carbs at breakfast is far more challenging. Sometimes your only option is a fruit cup, and sometimes even that comes drowned in simple syrup.

Airbnb is the anti-Four Seasons. Forget a front desk, doorman and porter. We picked up the key at a corner laundromat and let ourselves in to the first floor studio apartment. The place did not disappoint. It was light and clean. This was a huge relief as the biggest complaint people have using Airbnb is cleanliness.

The apartment had a small kitchen and a private garden. It was well stocked. We had no problem making eggs and bacon for breakfast. It even had wine glasses for an early evening drink in the garden. It was also filled with the owner's stuff. His diploma hung on the wall. Framed pictures of his girlfriend were placed strategically throughout. It was far less like staying in a hotel than it was borrowing an apartment from a friend. The owner also left us coffee and told us to "feel free to raid the liquor cabinet." The Four Seasons can't compete with that level of hospitality.

> **Fact:** Not every Airbnb experience is as positive as ours. One apartment we rejected had a review warning of mystery liquid dripping through the ceiling from the apartment above. Apparently, in the City, this is not exclusively an outdoor problem.

We had a fantastic trip, but we admit that it was not our most successful Drink Your Carbs vacation. We came back from the Las Vegas without gaining a single pound. New York, however, defeated our attempts to stick to our diet. This is odd, because navigating New York's food and drink scene while maintaining Drink Your Carbs should've been easy.

In New York restaurants, it's completely normal to modify an entrée to reduce the carbs and calories. When we ordered according to the Food List, no one reacted negatively. In fact, they offered suggestions for making items even healthier. Our cheating was never out of necessity. We simply got into a bad pattern of permissiveness. We could've just as easily stayed strict throughout.

> **Fact:** We did manage to eat a perfect DYC meal at Bier Craft, a beer garden and sandwich shop in Brooklyn. Along with the usual meats piled between slices of homemade bread, they had a "Paleo Jerk Chicken" on the menu. It was full half a chicken coated in jerk seasoning, served on top of bacon-filled collard greens and roasted broccoli. The dish was awesome, but it wasn't strictly Paleo. It would've been far more accurately described as "Drink Your Carbs Chicken."
>
> Loren Cordain, the author of the original Paleo Diet book, places both bacon and chicken thighs on his avoid list alongside bread and potatoes. He also limits beer to a single 12-ounce serving per day, which is challenging in a restaurant that serves pints.[2] (We added a footnote here because no adherent to the Paleo Diet would otherwise believe us.)

For every perfect Drink Your Carbs meal, however, we would break down and order some kind of starchy carb with the next. At Rare Bar and Grill, we ate amazing burger salads, but halfway through our meal broke down an ordered fries. At a small deli near the apartment, Steven ordered a breakfast sandwich on a poppy seed bagel two days in a row, while Andrea paired her scrambled eggs with home fries. This wouldn't have been a problem if we'd exercised or cut back on our drinking, but this isn't what happened. Our wine intake spiked as we spent our evenings drinking with friends and, during the 10-day trip, we worked out exactly twice.

This is not to say that the entire trip was a Drink Your Carbs disaster. The balance between our Drink Your Carbs meals and our cheats likely explains why neither of us came back five pounds heavier. For every meal that contained potatoes or lunch that contained French fries, we had at least one carb free banquet. Averaging our meals, our trip probably earned a solid C on Major Morgan's Grading Scale. It could've have been worse. But it also could've been far better.

There was no point in beating ourselves up over our dietary failures. Instead, we returned home and imposed our punishment: 10 days in Austerity Mode. We paid for our dietary transgressions by cleaning up our diet for the same number of days as we were travelling. It was a small price to pay for a fantastic vacation.

> **In Defense of Random Drips on New York Streets:** Neither of us returned home with mystery illness. Nor did we develop superpowers. Whatever it was that kept splashing us from above was evidently harmless.

Twenty Seven

Travel Case Study: Antarctica

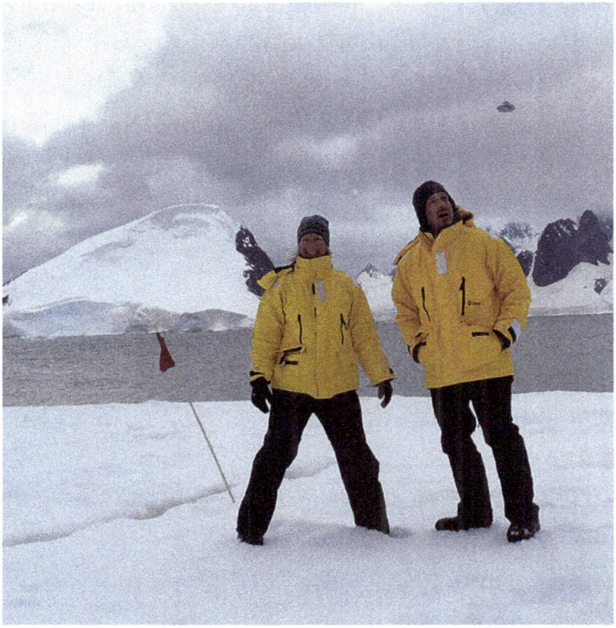

We took Drink Your Carbs to the bottom of the world to test it in one of the harshest environments on Earth.

While planning our expedition, we imagined ourselves as modern day Shackletons surviving only through a combination of wits, seal blubber and cask-strength whiskey.

As it turns out, this lifestyle is now prohibited under the Antarctic Treaty. These days, visiting is more like being transported into an episode of the *Love Boat* in which Puerto Vallarta has been replaced by a frozen continent. In our case, the role of Captain Stubing was played by a former Russian naval commander with a gruff demeanor that presumably concealed a heart of gold. Charo was played by a balding Canadian named Scott.

In other words, instead of hauling a wooden sledge through chest-deep snow, we did our trekking from a balcony suite on the Ocean Diamond, a Quark Expeditions luxury ship.

Antarctica is a hard place to describe and an even harder place to get to. It took three flights and nearly 20 hours in the air to travel from San Francisco to Ushuaia, a small city located at the tip of Argentina. From there we boarded the Ocean Diamond for a two-day sail across Drake's Passage.

Drake's Passage is one of the most feared stretches of open ocean on the planet. This is where the Pacific, Atlantic and Southern oceans meet, producing the kinds of ship-sinking swell that Hollywood spends millions of dollars recreating.

Since 1805, sailors have used the Beaufort scale to measure the relative fearsomeness of waves and wind. We prefer to compare our maritime conditions to rides at Disneyland. Our voyage from Argentina to Antarctica was abnormally serene; on our scale it ranked just below "It's a Small World."

Our return trip, however, was a different story. The Passage lived up to its stomach-turning reputation, throwing 25-foot waves at us alongside 89 mile-per-hour gusts. We liken that crossing to a car derailment on "Space Mountain" that sends you careening through the façade of "Cinderella's Castle." But we are getting ahead of ourselves.

Fact: The history of Antarctic exploration is largely a history of driving around looking for a place to park.

> Many early explorers were unable to set foot on the continent. Some were turned back by sea ice before they reached the Antarctic Circle. Others discovered long stretches of coast that were inaccessible; either the bays were clogged with icebergs or the coast itself consisted of an impenetrable 300-foot ice wall.
>
> Some of the early ninetieth century explorers returned home with detailed maps of mountains, islands and inlets that actually do not exist. Some historians blame poor navigation and inferior mapping skills. We believe the more likely explanation is that it was preferable to fabricate whole land masses than to report home having not claimed a single speck of rock for king and country.

We crossed the Antarctic Circle at 2 a.m. on our third night of sailing. An announcement went over the loudspeaker and we all gathered on the main deck for spiked hot chocolate and a deafening blast from the ship's horn.

We then spent the next few hours doing the maritime equivalent of circling the block. We tried every imaginable approach, but we could not push through the ice floes blocking access to Marguerite Bay.

There are days in San Francisco when we circle for parking for more than an hour before giving up and going home. Our captain ultimately made the same choice to turn back. By morning we had left the Circle behind and were motoring north along the Antarctic Peninsula.

Antarctica is an alien landscape. It is not, as we imagined, a frozen, featureless plateau. Jagged mountains run the entire length of the peninsula like blackened teeth jutting up through layers of ice and snow. Glaciers formed in these mountains terminate in icy cliffs along the shore.

For most of our journey, these brilliant blue and white cliffs stretched the entire length of the horizon. It was the vastness that impressed us most. The sheer enormity inspires the same sense of awe that comes from looking at stars on a perfectly clear night, far from lights of civilization. Or from driving on I-70 through Kansas.

Fact: We assumed that on our journey we would see stars further and brighter than we had ever seen before. We were wrong. The sun now sets on the British Empire, but it does not set in Antarctica during summertime. Around 10 p.m., the sun drops to the horizon producing the most colorful sunsets we have ever seen. The sun, however, never fully retreats. It continues pouring pinks, purples and reds into the surrounding landscape for hours before climbing back into the low sky.

If you come across a Match.com profile stating, "I love long walks, romantic dinners and three-hour sunsets," you now know where your suitor lives.

Adding to the alien nature of the landscape are huge icebergs carved by wind and water into sculptures as complex as anything on display in New York's Museum of Modern Art. We were lucky enough to see an iceberg roll over and we now know how the most remarkable shapes are formed. Thin spires and odd mushroom caps of ice form beneath the water as icebergs melt. Ultimately, this process leaves the icebergs top heavy forcing them to topple over to reveal these other-worldly shapes and contours.

Fact: Forget *March of the Penguins*. If you want to get a real sense of Antarctica, watch *The Empire Strikes Back*. Antarctica is a dead ringer for the rebel home world, Hoth. We spent the voyage half expecting an Imperial

Walker to peak over the snowy mountains and begin firing lasers at our ship.

More than one friend has asked, "Did you see polar bears?" The answer is no. We saw no bears because there are no bears to be seen. This is another example of something we should have researched before we left. We had no idea there are no native land mammals in Antarctica. On the bright side, we didn't have to embarrass ourselves by asking one of the guides. We figured it out the instant we saw a penguin waddling across the ice.

On land penguins are about as agile as one-year-old children. They wobble along like drunks, waving their little arms for balance. They frequently trip and fall. Had Charles Darwin visited the Antarctic instead of the Galapagos, the theory of evolution would surely include a chapter on nature's sense of humor. In the case of penguins, that sense of humor is distinctly slapstick.

Fact: There is no such thing as too many penguins.

Watching a penguin cross an ice floe, it is impossible not to appreciate the fact that penguins have no natural predators on land. Penguins are slow and clumsy on land because they can be. There is no advantage to moving faster or more gracefully. Simply put, penguins do not eat on land and nothing on land eats them. There are Skua, which are birds capable of taking a penguin chick, but Skua are too small to threaten full grown penguins. For penguins, land is home base.

It's a whole different story once they dive in the icy water. There, penguins are among the most agile creatures we have ever seen. This makes perfect sense when you consider that in water, penguins must be able to catch fish and krill. They also need to outrun or outmaneuver sharks, leopard seals and killer whales.

One of the great pleasures of the trip was watching penguins swim underneath our kayaks, darting and weaving like tiny fighter pilots. They are even more impressive when covering distance; they jump from the water like porpoises. They get serious air. On one of our ship's excursions, a penguin jumped into a Zodiac, landing in a woman's lap. Unfortunately, during the ensuing panic no one thought to snap a picture.

Fact: The only resident land mammals in Antarctica are humans. The first permanent human settlement was established in 1956.

According to Wikipedia, there are between 1,000 and 5,000 summertime residents scattered across the Antarctic continent.[1] According to Australia's Antarctic Research Division, this number dwindles to several hundred during the unending darkness of winter.[2] This presented a major problem for our plan to spread the message of Drink Your Carbs. There is virtually no one to spread it to. We met fewer than a dozen researchers who live on Antarctica. We interacted with them only briefly as we toured their facilities and shopped in their gift shops.

Fact: Vernadsky Station, one of two stations we visited, was built by the British in 1954. The base specializes in atmospheric research and is best known for taking the measurements that led to the discovery of the hole in the earth's ozone layer. Even more impressive than their scientific work, however, is the fact that directly above their laboratory sits a full bar as well stocked as any pub in London. That bar is the last stop on the Vernadsky tour.

It's not surprising that scientists working in one of the most remote places on earth would request the

> British government send materials to build a pub: bottles, taps, kegs, logoed mirrors, a brass rail and even a pool table. What amazes us is that some bureaucrat approved the expenditure and delivered the goods. As far as we are concerned, this was the last great act of the British Empire.
>
> Ukraine took over Vernadsky in 1991 and gave it its current name. The Ukrainians did not, however, change the bar. The only addition we could discern is that they now distill and flavor their own signature vodka.
>
> We raised our shot glasses. "To drinking our carbs in Antarctica."
>
> The two men behind the bar answered only "Nasdrovia."

It would turn out that those shots would be the only food or beverage we consumed on land. And, technically, Vernadsky is located on an island, so those shots may not qualify as drinking in Antarctica.

The Antarctic Treaty of 1959 was amended in 2004 to govern the behavior of tourists visiting the continent. The revised rules state that nothing may be left behind. This includes everything from bacteria—we dipped our boots in an antibacterial solution before venturing ashore—to trash, scraps of food or even human waste. In other words, no food or beverages other than water may come ashore and there is no ducking behind a rock to pee. We learned to dehydrate ourselves in advance of landing so that we would not have to return to the ship prematurely.

All of our dining took place on board the Ocean Diamond. From a Drink Your Carbs perspective, this meant that our challenge was staying on our diet on a luxury cruise liner rather than anything to do with being in a polar environment.

We spent only one night away from our heated cabin. On the sixth night of the voyage, we camped on the ice. We slept in bivy sacks, which are essentially full-body condoms into which you stuff yourself and your sleeping bag. It was cold and windy. The sun never set, so it was difficult to sleep. On the bright side, we were visited repeatedly by a pair of penguins whose territory we had clearly invaded.

Sleeping on the ice in Antarctica sounds tough, but the entire excursion lasted less than 10 hours. We were dropped off on a spit of ice around 9:30 in the evening and shuttled back to the ship for breakfast at 7 a.m. It felt less like camping and more like the time, back in high school, when we spent the night in a snowy parking lot to purchase U2 tickets.

Fact: Quark Expeditions truncated our camping trip for good reasons. The rules of Antarctica prohibited bringing ashore so much as a single protein bar. They had no choice but to drop us off after dinner.

Given the leave nothing rule, the simple act of relieving oneself was exceptionally complicated. Our expedition leaders built latrines from blocks of ice to give us a small measure of privacy, but the "toilets" had to comply with the Antarctic Treaty. They involved oversized buckets that were sealed in the morning and hauled back to the ship.

A few of our fellow campers found this immeasurably gross. Some people refused to go near them. The mere mention of them was enough to send one fellow guest reeling from the dinner table.

The upside of these restrictions, however, is that Antarctica is a truly pristine environment. There are

> very few signs of human intrusion. It is the only place we have ever been where we did not see even a single discarded candy wrapper or cigarette butt.

While we failed to spread the message of Drink Your Carbs to the Southern Continent, eating according to the rules of the Food List onboard the ship was simple. Breakfast consisted of eggs and bacon. Lunch was cobbled together from salads and proteins from a large buffet offering foods that we mostly could not eat. Dinner service was more formal and our waiter very quickly figured out that the best way to feed us was with plain grilled protein and steamed vegetables. It was by far our most successful Drink Your Carbs holiday. We both lost weight on the voyage.

Unfortunately, we cannot take full credit for our success. We very likely would have cheated more often had it been an option. For the first time in years, we were hamstrung by our food allergies. Over the past 20 years we have perfected ordering meals in restaurants that are wheat free, dairy free and still rich in flavor and complexity. Our secret lies in asking, "What do you think would be the best choice given our dietary afflictions?"

No matter how we asked that question, we receive the all too accommodating, "tell us what you want and the kitchen will prepare it." No matter what we ordered, the chef's solution was invariably to strip the dish of sauces and replace the sides with steamed vegetables. In other words, without any effort on our own part we found ourselves in Austerity Mode.

As we have mentioned, the downside of Austerity Mode is that it dramatically reduces calories and leaves you perpetually hungry. We ate until we were stuffed and 20 minutes later we were starving. While our fellow passengers whined about being overfed and gaining weight, we supplemented with the protein bars and beef jerky we always carry when we travel. By the third day of the cruise, we were obsessively counting and rationing our supplies. This was by far our most Shackleton-like experience.

"Is it just me, or are the penguins starting to look delicious?" Andrea asked near the end of the trip. It was not just her.

In fairness, we must note that the crew of the Ocean Diamond fed our fellow passengers like foie gras farms feed geese. Every few hours, more food was hauled from the kitchen. The main lounge served high tea complete with bottomless trays of cookies and cakes. The pre-dinner expedition meetings were paired with a buffet of deep fried nibbles. Late at night, the cookies and cakes reappeared. Because of our allergies, we ate exactly none of these.

We are not proud of this: the bulk of our between-meal calories came from the cocktail lounge. They had a respectable beer and wine selection, a few top shelf whiskeys and even a bottle of Amaro. From that list, we cobbled together the liquid lunch equivalent of between meal snacks.

> **Fact:** We came to refer to our pairing of Austerity Mode with slightly higher than reasonable alcohol consumption as "Party Mode." It is in no way an official part of the diet. But like the secret menu at In-N-Out Burger, it is available should a short-term need arise.

Maybe we didn't succeed in drinking our carbs on Antarctica, but we definitely consider the trip a resounding success. Antarctica is the first truly unspoiled landscape we have ever visited. We have climbed mountains. We have trekked into jungles. On this trip we got a small glimpse of what the world looks like with little to no human interference.

Equally remarkable was our ability to stick to our diet for the duration of a luxury cruise. Before we left we would've argued that it could not be done. We had plenty of help, but we nonetheless feel that we accomplished something just short of miraculous. It was so successful that we just booked another Quark cruise to the Arctic.

The best part of our upcoming Arctic itinerary is that the entire trip takes place in protected waters. There will be no repeat of our second crossing of Drake's Passage. Even our Captain remarked that the crossing was one of the worse of the year. Waves crested over the deck and drenched windows on the seventh floor. The ship listed so severely that lunch dishes skittered off the buffet and shattered against a far wall. Most of our fellow passengers were too sick to leave their staterooms.

Our Arctic cruise will, almost assuredly, take place in waters no rougher than the ride through Disney's "Haunted Mansion."

Also, for the Arctic, we will bring more snacks. This way Steven should never have to ask, "Is it just me, or are the polar bears starting to look delicious?"

Twenty Eight

Travel Case Study: Middle East

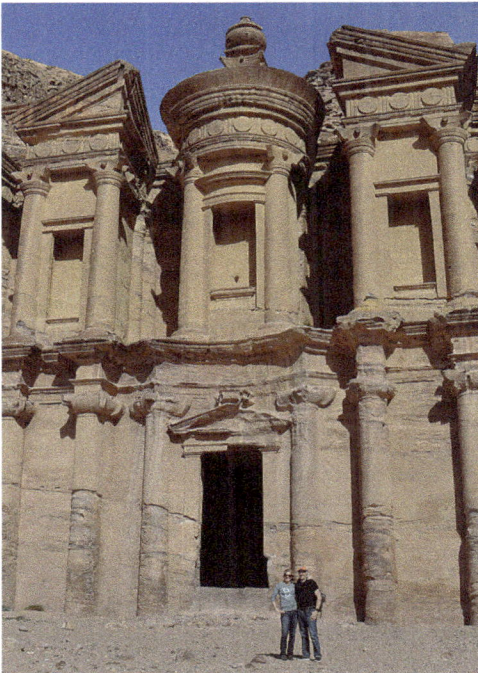

This dispatch comes straight from the First Class cabin of an Air Canada jet on route from Tel Aviv, Israel to Toronto, Canada. We mention our class of service only because anyone who has taken this flight will know just how much this upgrade means. Somewhere in the back of the plane, some poor fool is sandwiched between a crying child in the middle seat and men in black suits praying audibly in the aisle.

On this particular flight, a half dozen members of the ultra-orthodox Lubavitch sect of Judaism are currently deep in prayer, blocking access to the bathroom at the back of the plane. We rejected the idea of heading back there to tell them that they're praying in the wrong direction. There's no chance they'll believe us even though we're right. The problem is that the men are operating under the misconception that because we are flying away from Israel, Jerusalem is behind us. Religious Yeshivas might do well to cut a few hours of Talmud in favor of explaining the geometry behind great circles. For those who have forgotten, great circles explain why it is, when circumnavigating a ball, the shortest path between two points often requires you to head due north. At this point in the flight, these men should now be facing the left side of the hull. As things stand, they are praying to the suburbs south of Moscow.

Staying on Drink Your Carbs, like everything else in Israel, is complicated. Breakfast was easy. Whereas a standard American hotel buffet offers an entire lineup of greasy potatoes and breakfast meats, an Israeli breakfast buffet includes a world-class salad bar with dozens of choices including diced cubes of tomato and cucumber, shredded herbs tossed in lemon juice and usually some form of pickled cabbage and beets swimming in mayonnaise tinted the color of Pepto-Bismol. The lettuce was fresh. The vegetables were crisp. There were the ubiquitous tables of breakfast pastries and an omelet station for the tourists, but the locals clearly favored fresh salads, pickled fish and goat cheese. The best way to understand the typical Israeli breakfast buffet is to imagine a high-speed crash between a raw food restaurant and a Kosher Assisted Living Facility.

In Drink Your Carbs terms, lunch and dinner were as difficult as breakfast was easy. Finding an Israeli lunch that does not come wrapped in a pita is like digging a hole in that country without finding something of archeological significance. It happens, but it's rare. The pita conundrum took a particularly heavy toll on Andrea who, as we have mentioned, is allergic to wheat.

Her typical lunch involved meat and hummus eaten either with a spoon or, in flagrant violation of the Food List, scooped up on French fries. Steven took a different approach: he violated every dietary principal he held sacred and scarfed down pita, lafa (really big pita) and tortilla-like Druze bread with a reckless abandon the Holy Land hasn't seen since the Romans were expelled.

A brief note on the topic of hummus: We in America have long viewed hummus as a topping or side dish. Hummus would never be the focal point of a meal. It usually serves as an alternative to chips and salsa. It turns out that our marginalization of hummus has nothing to do with culinary tradition. It turns out that our hummus just sucks. We never knew this because, as Americans, we can only compare our hummus to itself. There are hummus joints in Israel that are—and we do not say this lightly—life changing.

Hummus Kitchen on Nahalat Binyamin Street in Tel Aviv serves bowls of hummus topped with a choice of mushrooms, lamb, eggplant, falafel or tahini. It didn't matter that Andrea was forced to eat it with a spoon while Steven was able to dip into it with pita so fresh it was still baking in the basket on the table. It was among the best foods either of us has ever tasted. It was nothing like hummus back home. The richness and subtlety is indescribable. No amount of wishing will make it otherwise: American hummus is the equivalent of 7-Eleven sushi.

Dinners in Israel varied wildly and varied largely based on the ancient laws of kashrut. Most of the restaurants in Israel are strictly kosher. This means they cleave to an exhaustive set of rules for food preparation, the most obvious and impactful of which is milk and meat cannot be served in the same meal. As a result, kosher restaurants serve either dairy or meat. A few kosher restaurants serve both, but in order to do so they maintain separate kitchens and use a divider to split the dining room. Unless you are prepared to talk to the other people in your party exclusively through text messaging, you still have to choose between meat and milk.

Oddly, fish is considered neither meat nor milk and as a result can be served in any kosher restaurant. Fish, under the laws of kashrut, are classified as parve, the same category as broccoli and carrots. And, as if the rules did not seem arbitrary enough, chicken and other poultry are meat but eggs are parve like fish. The laws of kashrut definitely make more sense to people who grew up with them. To those of us who did not grow up in kosher households, they seem completely random.

It is also worth mentioning that the restrictions of kashrut have been embraced by Israeli chefs as more of a challenge than a handicap. These chefs have mastered poultry product smoked and dyed to imitate both the look and taste of pork. They have also taken non-dairy desserts to a height that we would have thought impossible. We have no idea how they do it, but we suppose that this is to be expected after 5,000 years of practice.

The separation of milk and meat posed an interesting challenge. Dairy restaurants tend to add dairy to everything they serve. Since Steven is allergic to all forms of milk, eating in these restaurants left him with few options beyond the salad course. More than once, Steven was forced to grab a falafel on the way back to the hotel after dinner.

Andrea had similar difficulties with meat restaurants. Israeli cuisine tends to be wheat heavy. Meat restaurants are even more so. On most meat menus, Andrea had one choice. Everything else was either breaded or lightly floured before cooking. It didn't help that neither of us is a huge fan of kosher steak. The koshering process involves salting the meat to draw out all of the blood. The process is perfect for ground meat, sausage and anything else that will be spiced and chopped into bits. With steaks, however, bloodletting yields a consistency akin to chewing gum. Apparently God prefers beef to be the texture of calamari—which is theologically fascinating considering that calamari is not kosher.

In meat restaurants, Andrea stuck largely to fish when it was not breaded and, at times, cobbled together a dinner from a couple of appetizers. Steven, as we said, went crazy. There is nothing in a meat restaurant Steven cannot eat. There are no dairy products in the kitchen. If someone were to so much as bring in a cup of coffee with cream, the entire kitchen would have to be scrubbed clean and inspected by a rabbi. Our guess is that if you found a rat in a kosher kitchen, the remediation process would not be as severe. So, for Steven, it was the first time in years where he could literally order anything and everything on the menu. While Andrea looked on, Steven got to try 1,000 forms of beef and lamb wrapped in flaky filo dough.

Steven definitely played fast and loose with the Food List, but Andrea was also unable to completely adhere. The problem was too many desserts. Let us be clear that we never once ordered dessert. We prefer our dessert to come in the form of an additional glass of wine. However, it turns out that Israelis, despite what you might have heard, are some of the nicest people on earth. It was almost impossible to escape from a dinner without being presented with a custom-made, wheat-free dairy-free sweet. We made a point of sharing with the rest of the people at our table, but politeness demanded that we consume far more sugar than we would have under normal circumstances.

There is a third choice in Israeli cuisine beyond milk and meat: treyf. Treyf is the Yiddish term for anything non-kosher. A treyf restaurant will serve cheeseburgers, shellfish and even pork. In Jerusalem, treyf is hard to find. In Tel Aviv and other larger cities, treyf may actually dominate. And there's no question that Israel does treyf as well as any country in the world. By far our best meal was at Herbert Samuel, a "high treyf" bistro in Tel Aviv. This restaurant would be just as crowded if it were located in San Francisco.

Herbert Samuel felt naughty after two weeks in Israel. Although we don't eat kosher at home, after two weeks of eating according to the rules of kashrut the oyster appetizer took on an air of forbidden pleasure. The oysters were served with a raw quail egg and a wasabi avocado puree. It's a preparation we hope that restaurants in our neighborhood will steal. They were spectacular. And eating them in Israel made them even better. The dish combined a world-class preparation with the mindless adrenalin of teenage rebellion.

The downside of a treyf restaurant became apparent when we were accidentally served a steak swimming in butter. Andrea ate the steak and says it was one of the best she has ever eaten. Steven was forced to watch from the sidelines. The kitchen did, however, bring him an incredible sashimi plate as both dinner and an apology. Even with the butter snafu, the meal was as good as any we have had anywhere in the world.

Overall, we found incredible respect for our dietary restrictions. It wasn't always easy, but it turns out that people who can handle the rules of kashrut can easily manage our peccadillos. Dairy restaurants were harder for Steven and meat restaurants were harder for Andrea, but in all cases Israelis were incredibly helpful in steering us towards food that met our allergy restrictions. Staying on Drink Your Carbs, however, was another matter altogether. Israel is just not the place to avoid simple carbs; they are too good and too deeply embedded into Israeli cuisine. As Drink Your Carbs continues to spread, we hope more options will be added which follow the rigors of our Food List. Until then, we recommend that anyone headed to this part of the Middle East spend some time in Austerity Mode in advance of the trip. Earn your pita before you leave so your hummus can be enjoyed guilt free.

It should come as no surprise that between kosher dairy, kosher meat and outright treyf, treyf restaurants were our favorite. Some day we will venture to the back of the plane to ask the gentlemen currently praying to Iceland, "If God did not want us to eat pork and shellfish, why did he make them so delicious?"

Twenty Nine

Travel Case Study: Crete, Greece

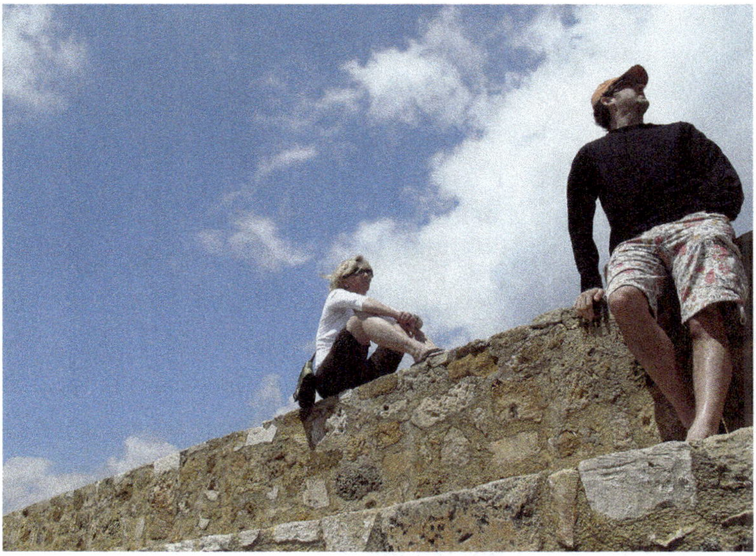

We are adventurous eaters. Aside from a few obvious restrictions from allergies and Drink Your Carbs, pretty much anything else is fair game. If we're travelling and the local delicacy is squirrel heads our only question is: "How are they prepared?" As long as they aren't battered, fried or drowned in a cream sauce, we're all over it.

Of all of the foods we've been fortunate to try, the most perfect Drink Your Carbs food we have ever come across was Meat

Cooked in the Manner of Thieves on the Greek island of Crete. Whole, salted fish-on-a-stick in Kyoto, Japan was a close second, but it just can't compete when it comes to backstory.

> **Fact:** We took this trip four years ago. At the time, Greece had no riots. The economy was weak, but there was an overwhelming sense of optimism in everyone we met. The Euro crisis changed all that. Greece of today is a far angrier place. We mention this to explain why the Greece we recall sounds very different from the one pictured on the news. Without this context, it might sound as though we skipped traveling all the way to Europe and instead swung by the souvlaki stand at Epcot Center.

We have mentioned before that renting an apartment or villa is by far the easiest way to travel on Drink Your Carbs. If you have a kitchen, you can shop for local meat and cook you own healthy, low-carb meals. We certainly don't recommend cooking all of your own meals. You need to get out and explore the local fare. However, being able to fully control even one meal a day makes a huge difference in limiting your dietary damage.

> **Fact:** While visiting London a few years ago, we were served deep-fried toast under the name "Typical English Breakfast." We have no idea how throwing slices of white bread into a deep fryer became typically English. All we know is that, unbelievably, there exists a less Drink Your Carbs breakfast option than the typical American breakfast of hash browns and big stacks of pancakes.

Our rented villa was a big house on the edge of the town of Meladoni with four bedrooms, a large kitchen and two living rooms. The walled garden was full of fresh herbs and orange trees laden with fruit. A huge barbeque grill dominated one side of the house and a modest, but beautifully maintained, swimming pool sat on the other. If not for the fact that the weather was unseasonably cold, the pool would have been perfect for dips in the late afternoon after we'd returned home from touring the island. Instead of swimming, our afternoons were spent huddled around the barbeque for heat as we drank Raki and prepared grilled dinners of various local meats.

Fact: Raki is most certainly the official drink of Crete. Raki is a liquor as clear as vodka and as rough drinking as a shot of rubbing alcohol. It's distilled from grapes, although it's less grappa than moonshine. In defense of Raki, the more you drink the easier it goes down. And, in an emergency, it could probably run a car.

As far as we could tell, every family on Crete distills their own Raki. After a family's grapes are pressed into wine, the remaining skins and seeds are distilled to rescue any lingering alcohol. Raki is not aged. The moment it drips from the still, it's ready to drink.

Raki seems almost designed for Drink Your Carbs. Raki is always served straight up, at room temperature. No matter how unpalatable a given batch might be, it's never blended or sweetened. The No Mixer Rule has been in effect on Crete for centuries.

We were served Raki everywhere we went. It showed up in small pitchers after every lunch and dinner. It was served by shopkeepers to thank us for making

> purchases. It was offered every time we were invited into someone's home. If you ask, there is Raki available for purchase at every gas station, supermarket, bakery, butcher shop, vegetable stand and even the occasional sandal shop. We bought one bottle that was made by the Monks at the Monastery of Aghia-Irin. In spite of the fact that the Monks have been perfecting their recipe since the 14th century, it was by far the hairiest bottle we purchased and was the only bottle we could not finish.

One concern about cooking too many meals in your villa is that you might be tempted to prepare the same foods you eat at home and miss some of the local flavors and specialties.

On Crete, this would not be possible. Even a food as common as chicken is very different when bought in a Cretan butcher shop. In America, we expect our meat to be unidentifiable as to the original animal. Our steaks look nothing like cows. Our chops and ribs are stacked and uniform so as to avoid looking pig or lamb-like. Even chickens are tucked and trimmed until they barely evoke images of fowl.

Cretan chickens look as though they have been little more than de-feathered. The heads are removed, but the long neck is left fully attached and intact, as are most of the internal organs within the chicken's cavity. But what really separates Cretan chicken from the chicken we've grown accustomed to in America is the butchering technique.

We visited three separate butcher shops while on the island, so we know that the butchering we saw was not limited to a single individual or store. It works like this: first, the neck is hacked off with a large wooden-handled cleaver and the fleshy tube that is the detached neck is set off to the side. The body of the chicken is then carefully bisected down the middle. That was the only part of the process we found familiar. Once the halves are separated, both are subjected to brutal treatment.

Instead of being carefully dismembered into individual breasts, thighs and legs, they are cleaved apart into random chunks. Picture Norman Bates hacking apart Janet Leigh in the movie Psycho. Now replace Norman's knife with a heavy meat cleaver, the shower with a large butchers block and Ms. Leigh with half a chicken laying cut side down. Even the sound screams low budget horror. Whack! Whack! Whack! The practice produces unpredictable pieces of commingled white and dark meat. Also, bone shards that must be picked from your teeth like buckshot from a hunted pheasant.

The treatment of pork and lamb must be equally violent. We bought already prepared chops and ribs from the refrigerated case, and while they looked similar to meat we might have bought at home, the splintering of the bones indicated a less-than-gentle process. There are very few cows on Crete and we never saw beef sold, but we assume that butchering a cow Cretan-style would involve a jackhammer.

The meat on Crete is among the absolute best we have ever tasted. Chicken, goats and lambs run free on the hillsides. Animals graze on wild onions and oregano that grow everywhere like weeds. The animals are marinating themselves from within. It is a complete mystery as to why such wonderful meat is subjected to such primitive butchering.

> **Case Study in Cretan Butchering:** One evening, toward the end of our trip, we served an irregularly shaped piece of grilled chicken breast to our friend and traveling companion, Tricia. Tricia is at best a reluctant meat eater. She prefers white meat that in no

way resembles the animal it came from. We examined every piece of the chicken we had grilled and served her the most benign-looking piece.

Half way through eating it, she flipped her chicken over. Still attached to underside of the breast was the chicken's lung. It was wrinkly and pink and looked like a deflated balloon.

Three questions remain unanswered:

1. Why is it that the lung is always served to the person least able to cope with it?
2. Is it possible that finding a lung in your chicken is lucky, like finding the plastic baby in a New Orleans king cake?
3. Why was the lung still wet and pink when it really should have been cooked to gray?

While grilling outside on the open-air barbeque, we had been drinking liberal quantities of Raki. Perhaps the whole incident can be blamed on a combination of moonlight and moonshine.

Another concern of renting a villa or apartment is that it can limit the time that is spent mingling with locals. Evenings spent in the villa or afternoons lounging by the pool might otherwise have been spent in restaurants or bars or even just wandering the streets of an unfamiliar city. Once again, this was not a problem on Crete. Not only did we meet a ton of locals, we were adopted by a Cretan family who brought us home for Easter dinner.

On past trips, most of our socializing with locals took place at night in pubs. The closest thing the town of Meladoni has to a pub is the old men who gather around plastic tables at the local Shell station to drink Raki alongside the gas pumps. We'll never know how the local gas station became a community gathering point. We never stopped to ask or to see if they would pour us a drink. The scene was not particularly inviting. It was all men. They were all dressed head-to-toe in black. They glared suspiciously each time we passed. Their behavior would make a lot more sense if it turned out that they weren't just drinking socially, but rather planning a bank heist.

We didn't meet the family who adopted us in a local bar. We met them during Easter services. The friends we were travelling with regularly attend church. The last time we went to church was 17 years ago during our honeymoon in Venice, Italy. We woke up early one morning to attend Mass in St. Mark's Basilica. The woman who ran the youth hostel where we were staying woke up even earlier than we did in order to brew coffee and make us breakfast. She did this out of respect for the fact that we were obviously very religious. We didn't have the heart to tell her that we actually just wanted to see the Basilica without waiting in a two-hour line.

On the evening of Good Friday, we found ourselves standing in front of a beautiful church in the center of Meladoni. Crete was in the middle of an unusual cold spell. We could see our breath against the clear black sky. Families streamed in and out of the church. Inside, we could hear priests chanting. The question that kept us frozen in the courtyard was, "Is it okay for people who aren't Greek Orthodox to go inside?" Luckily, that question was overheard by a local woman who answered us in a perfect Long Island accent, "You're welcome in any church in Greece."

Inside the church, priests chanted from behind a screen, out of sight. Worshipers lit candles and placed them in boxes on either side of the altar. As the boxes filled up, an old man stepped forward to scoop handfuls of candles out of the boxes and extinguish them in a bowl of water. As if to prove that the universe has a sense of humor, the man whose job it was to extinguish the flames of the faithful looked a lot like the late Christopher Hitchens.

The crowd was not particularly quiet, reverent or attentive. People talked and laughed. Children played right up until the moment that the priests came out from behind the screens to conclude the service. Suddenly, a hush fell over room. Everyone who was still in the courtyard pushed his or her way inside. Children who moments before were chasing one another through the crowd now stood reverently at their parent's feet.

We filed out of the Church after the service to be greeted by a 10-foot column of flames. While it was a shock, we should have seen this coming. While standing in the courtyard we noticed teenagers piling wood in the middle of the narrow street that ran alongside the church. We were completely mystified as to why local kids would stack logs on the evening of Good Friday, but we were too timid to ask. It became clear the moment we saw the bonfire.

Flames reached nearly as high as the church steeple. It must have been visible for miles around. Oddly, we seemed to be the only people concerned about flames leaping to nearby buildings or lapping at the overhead power lines.

Fact: The risks involved in igniting a huge bonfire on a narrow street in the middle of town paled in comparison to what occurred after services the next night. At the end of Midnight Mass, after the priest recited the words "Christos Anesti (Christ has risen)," men ran from the church to fire guns into the air. One man pulled an Uzi from beneath his leather jacket and unloaded a magazine in a matter of seconds. People inside the church and in the courtyard cheered the chaos.

> While Good Friday bonfires are a tradition throughout Greece, greeting the resurrection with gunfire is Crete-specific. The tradition is made all the more Cretan by the fact that most firearms are banned by the European Union. Cretans have a reputation for being fiercely independent. No regulatory subcommittee in Brussels is about to change that.

The night ended with a candlelit procession through town. It was during this ritual that we were adopted. As the orange glow of the bonfire faded, baskets of candles and a large wooden cross were brought from the church. The candles were distributed and lit. Young men then hoisted the cross above their heads and led us on a procession through Melidoni. As we walked, the family we had been talking to before the service invited us back to their house for "café" which turned out to be a euphemism for wine.

Their home was over 300 years old. It had passed through the generations. They were the only family ever to occupy it. The floors were originally dirt. There was no electricity or indoor plumbing and the sole source of heating was a large stone fireplace.

Over the years, the house had been repeatedly updated and was completely modern. Yet they managed to preserve much of the original details and character. The original stones of the walls still formed archways above the windows and doors. The centuries old fireplace still stood as the centerpiece of the kitchen. The combination of old and new was stunning.

> **Fact:** According to the World Health Organization, Greece has the most cigarette smokers per capita in the European Union.[1] According to an Oxford University survey, Crete has the highest percentage of smokers in Greece.[2]

> The Cretan attitude towards smoking was summed up by one of our hosts. He took a long drag off a cigarette and blew the smoke toward the stone fireplace. "The EU says that we are not allowed to smoke in enclosed spaces, not even in our own homes. But this is Crete. Would anyone else like a cigarette?"

By the end of the evening, we were invited to Easter dinner. It took place in the family's farmhouse at the bottom of a deep valley, down a long dirt road. There were ample reminders that this was a working farm. The family's goats and sheep roamed the grassy hillsides above. A nearby enclosure housed chickens and pigs. The farmhouse itself predated the house in town by nearly a century. It was constructed from stacked and mortared grey stones. It had been a ruin when the family acquired the land. It had been lovingly restored to serve as home base for family celebrations. No one lived there. There were no bedrooms. Most of the house was occupied by a wooden table long enough to serve three generations of family and invited guests.

The main course was the most perfect Drink Your Carbs entrée ever conceived. On the surface it looked like roasted lamb. Roasting lamb on a hand-turned rotisserie is traditional throughout Greece. However, our family had a slightly different culinary practice that took roasted lamb and gave it a Drink Your Carbs twist.

The patriarch of the family was, in his youth, one of the greatest poachers in all of Crete. He stole animals from shepherds all over the island, the family informed us with no shortage of pride. For years he remained at large, despite strong suspicion regularly cast in his direction. The problem was that no one could ever catch him in the act. The secret to his success, he told us, was that he only stole to eat. He never kept or sold a stolen animal.

The moment livestock was in his possession he would gather friends and feast. Long before the sun came up, the evidence had been eaten.

Eventually his luck ran out and he was thrown in jail. When that did nothing to deter him, he was exiled for several years from the island. For the record, he is now an upstanding citizen. From his time as Crete's leading poacher, however, he became an accidental world-class chef.

Instead of roasting an animal whole on a hand-turned spit, our outlaw hero butchered the animal onto multiple skewers that were then perched in a ring around the outside of a campfire. His reasons were twofold: meat cooks faster in smaller pieces and faster is better when trying not to get caught. More importantly, the skewers were positioned outside the campfire, rather than being locked into a rotisserie. If the owner of the animal happened along, the patriarch and his friends could each grab a skewer and run in separate directions. One of them might be caught, but they'd never get all of them.

Meat cooked in the manner of thieves is healthy, low carb and protein rich. The animals they procured were pasture-raised, filled with healthy fats and free of hormones. But this is true of all meat raised on Crete. What separates meat cooked in the manner of thieves is that it is designed to grab and run. While we never saw anyone racing across a hillside swinging a smoking skewer, the fact that the cooking method anticipates this behavior is enough for us to declare it as the most perfect Drink Your Carbs food in the world.

There is one small downside to cooking meat in the manner of thieves. Cooking the meat evenly is exceedingly difficult. Managing one skewer on a turn crank is simple. Managing five skewers that must be rotated by hand is another matter.

Most of the meat was cooked perfectly. It was crisp on the

outside, tender within. Andrea did, however, come across one piece that was at the extreme end of rare. The moment she exposed the pink meat, one of the older women at the table grabbed her by the wrist and said, "Don't eat that. That one's still running up the hillside."

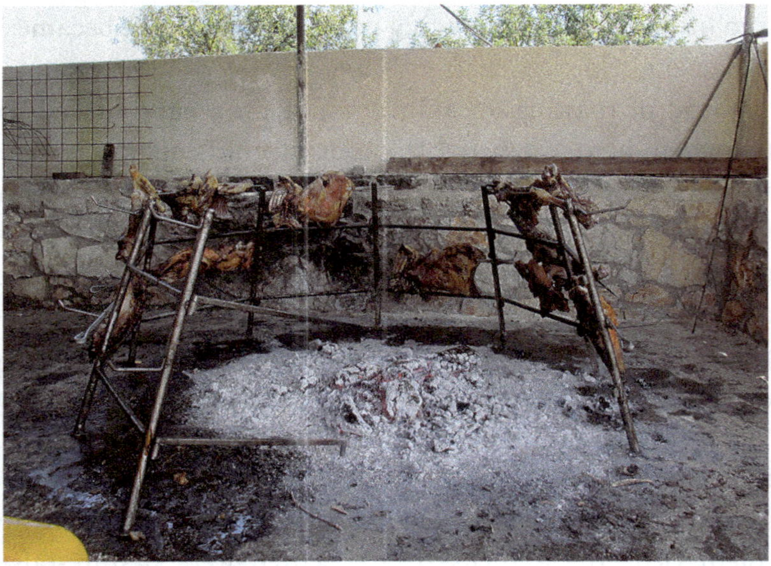

Thirty

Case Study

"Drink Your Carbs is so much more enjoyable than actual dieting."
—Dirk, Denver, Colorado

When Steven first told Dirk about Drink Your Carbs, they were having lunch at a Denver sushi restaurant. The sun was shining and the sky was a deep, cloudless blue. In bright daylight, Dirk's haggard, worn-out and generally gray appearance was even more evident. Dirk's wife had just given birth to their first child. Dirk hadn't slept through the night for nearly two months. He was clearly happy, but his excitement at being a new father was wrapped in a cloak of exhaustion.

Every father we know put on weight in the months leading up to and following the birth of his child. This is hardly unusual. After the birth of a child, family and friends come to visit bearing lasagna, cookies, cakes and other delicious, high-calorie foods of celebration. Going out for a run or doing any other exercise becomes the lowest priority. Gaining weight in the wake of a birth is typical, but even by those standards Dirk was extreme. Over the course of lunch, Dirk confessed that since the baby was born he had gained more than 20 pounds. Over the same period of time, the baby, whose only job at that point in his life was to grow and gain weight, put on about four.

Dirk had the 1970s childhood that BuzzFeed makes annoying lists about, including breakfasts consisting of Cookie Crisp cereal eaten in front of Saturday morning cartoons. In many ways, it was similar to Steven's. They both picked cereal based on the prize inside the box. They both had a weakness for strawberry-flavored Quik milk. They both worshiped anything and everything produced by Hostess. (Note that we didn't say "baked" because we have no idea how the raw ingredients and chemicals are combined to form a Twinkie.)

In both households, dessert was a birthright, not a treat. Think about it—if you're eating chocolate chip cookies for breakfast, you really think a parent will deny you an ice cream after dinner? The biggest difference was that Dirk's mother worked at Safeway. As a result, every can of soda he drank and every box of Little Debbie Snack Cakes he opened came home already dented or crushed.

The likely reason Dirk was not overweight as a child—and this holds true for Steven as well—is that both of them spent huge amounts of time running around outside. There is strong evidence that the current childhood obesity epidemic can be at least partially blamed on sedentary activities such as watching television and playing video games.[1] Whereas Dirk and Steven ran around the neighborhood with friends, today's kids interact while sitting still, staring straight forward.

Dirk played on his school's football and baseball teams and, in the off-season, he ran on his own. Through college and beyond, whenever his weight began to rise, he increased his mileage and reversed the trend. Until his son was born, that strategy had never failed him.

Then everything changed. With all of his energy devoted to caring for his wife and newborn son, Dirk stopped running. At the same time, his diet shifted dramatically. Every time he woke up during the night, and headed down to the kitchen to get his wife a glass of water and a snack, he would grab himself a bite of cake or a couple of cookies. As Dirk himself pointed out, "Every time my son had a nightly feeding, I also fed myself."

When Dirk heard about Drink Your Carbs over sushi that afternoon, he visibly brightened. Dirk is by no mean a heavy drinker, but he enjoys a beer or glass of wine with dinner or at the end of a long day. He assumed that if he wanted to lose weight, that ritual would have to be abandoned. Steven assured him that this was not the case.

At that time, Drink Your Carbs was very much in its infancy. The Food List did not yet exist. Drink Your Carbs consisted solely of three simple rules: Avoid simple carbs. No added sugar. Stay away from all things deep-fried.

Dirk took those rules home and became the first person, apart from Steven and Andrea, to be a test subject in this brand new approach to dieting.

Over the three months following that fateful lunch, human test subject Dirk lost all of the weight he'd gained. His weight has remained stable for over five years since. Whenever his weight fluctuates, which it invariably does around vacations and family holidays, he simply rededicates himself to Drink Your Carbs. "Sometimes I'm more relaxed with my diet. Other times I go through weeks without a single M&M."

Steven spoke with Dirk recently, just after the birth of his second child. Dirk is still running, still trim and still living on Drink Your Carbs. Last year he completed the New York Marathon.

"Beyond health benefits, there is the psychological benefit of knowing I can still drink," he said. "I find it easier to stick to both working out and eating well knowing I can have a couple of drinks with dinner."

Simply put, Dirk lives Drink Your Carbs and it works.

Thirty One

A History of Drinker's Diets

When we created Drink Your Carbs we assumed that ours was the first diet designed specifically for people who wanted to lose weight while continuing to drink alcohol. We were wrong by 150 years.

The first drinker's diet was published in 1863 under the title *Letter on Corpulence, Addressed to the Public.*[1] The author was a British mortician named William Banting. The entire diet is less than 20 pages long. Actual advice for weight loss takes up less than two of those pages. The rest of the letter is dedicated to Banting whining about his various physical ailments. Reading it feels a lot like visiting your grandfather in a rest home.

Banting began his book in wonderfully overstated fashion. "Of all the parasites that affect humanity I do not know of, nor can I imagine, any more distressing than that of obesity," he wrote.

Eventually, and after much hyperbole, Banting finally describes his diet. Banting's restrictions should sound familiar to anyone who has read a diet book written in the past two decades: no "bread, butter, milk, sugar, beer, and potatoes."

In 1863, these recommendations were considered radical. The medical establishment had a conniption and universally panned the diet as outright dangerous. Today, we can see the Banting recommendations for what they are, a relatively standard low-carb program.

Banting pairs his food restrictions with a drinking regimen that would incapacitate most normal humans, including a cordial with breakfast, wine with lunch, wine with dinner and a nightcap of "[a] tumbler or grog—(gin, whisky, or brandy, without sugar)—or a glass or two of claret or sherry." Not only did Banting create the first drinker's diet, his "without sugar" requirement is unquestionably the original prototype of our No Mixers rule.

The mere description of the quantity of alcohol Banting drank on a daily basis gives us a hangover. This is the reason Drink Your Carbs requires exercise. It would be virtually impossible to follow to the letter the Banting diet and still make it to your morning workout. This should be sufficient reason not to "Bant," as the diet was referred to in its day.

> **Fact:** The strangest thing in *Letter on Corpulence* is Banting's repeated recommendation that dieters consume large quantities of toast on a diet that prohibits bread. Stranger still is Banting's reason: "I feel certain [bread] is more wholesome if thoroughly toasted."

The second drinker's diet before Drink Your Carbs was also published in the form of a pamphlet. In 1964, Robert Cameron published *The Drinking Man's Diet: How to Lose Weight with a Minimum of Will Power.*[2] Strangely, Cameron wrote the book under two pseudonyms, Gardner Jameson and Elliott Williams. Perhaps Cameron thought that listing multiple authors would add intellectual heft to a diet he is able to explain in two sentences: "Eat less than 60 grams of carbohydrates a day. That's all there is to it."

Like Banting's diet, Cameron's diet was not without controversy. In 1965, Time Magazine reviewed the diet and concluded that "*The Drinking Man's Diet* is utter nonsense, has no scientific basis, and is chock-full of errors. . . . [I]f a man eats and drinks heavily, he is going to gain weight and get drunk."[3]

We agree with Time Magazine that Cameron's pamphlet is filled with errors. Cameron lists wine as having no carbohydrates and Mint Juleps—a classic Southern cocktail that contains enough sugar to make a can of Dr. Pepper seem savory by comparison—as having only three.

We take issue with the rest of the Time review. The review attempts to make the argument that alcohol consumption is incompatible with dieting. It minces no words. "The book's contents are a cocktail of wishful thinking, a jigger of nonsense and a dash of sound advice." We have spent years working to prove that this assertion is not true.

Aside from the mathematical errors, *The Drinking Man's Diet* is impressive both for its simplicity and effectiveness. We have no doubt that if someone can really hold themselves to 60 grams of carbohydrates a day, they will lose weight. A limit of 60 grams of carbohydrates effectively removes all sugars and starches from a person's diet. The result will be calorie restriction and weight loss, even without any recommendations for exercise. This is, of course, assuming that they don't rely on Cameron's fuzzy math for the carb counts.

It is also worth noting that under the heading "Scientific Basis," Cameron cites Banting's weight loss as proof of the effectiveness of *The Drinking Man's Diet*. It's never a good sign when an author has to go back 101 years to dig up a success story.

Fact: Citing Banting is odd, but it's not the strangest thing in *The Drinking Man's Diet*. That would be the

> recommendation that we all eat plenty of Raccoon, Opossum and Whale. (Odder still is the fact that he categorizes all three as "Poultry.") We didn't even bother to add Raccoon or Opossum to the Drink Your Carbs Food List. In this particular case, we agree with Mr. Cameron that roadkill should be unlimited. But being a decidedly less manly diet, we didn't see the need to bring it up.
>
> While we agree that Opossum and Raccoon can be enjoyed in limitless quantities, we part ways with Cameron on the consumption of Whale. We have said this before and we stand by it: if it's on the endangered species list it's not on Drink Your Carbs. There is no exception to this rule. Until the U.S. Department of Fish and Wildlife removes all species of whales from the list, it's off the menu.

The most recent drinker's diet, *The Drunk Diet: How I Lost 40 Pounds . . . Wasted,* was published in 2012.[4] We noticed it, but we never picked up a copy because everything we read about it described it as a memoir rather than a diet. Every reviewer focused on the fact that the author, Lüc Carl, was an ex-boyfriend of Lady Gaga. And none of the reviews we saw bothered to mention that the book contained a serious diet and exercise plan. Until Carl reached out to us on Twitter, we assumed *The Drunk Diet* was a celebrity tell-all wrapped in a misleading but otherwise awesome title.

Comparing *The Drunk Diet* to Drink Your Carbs is like comparing Hunter S. Thompson's *Fear and Loathing in Las Vegas* to the *Lonely Planet Guide to Las Vegas.* Both books touch on local landmarks, but the similarities end there. *The Drunk Diet* is written for people who want to channel their inner Lindsay

Lohan and party like rock stars. Drink Your Carbs is for people who enjoy ordering drinks with dinner and throwing back beers at a baseball game. While DYCers occasionally swallow instead of spit at a wine tasting, it's rare to see us up past midnight.

> **Fact:** *The Drunk Diet* is a hard book to describe. Imagine throwing a traditional diet book into a blender along with Keith Richards' new autobiography, a pair of tight leather pants and a shitload of hair-care products. *The Drunk Diet* reads like that smoothie would taste.

The Drunk Diet tells the story of Lüc Carl growing up in the Midwest, playing in heavy metal bands and hanging out with meth addicts.

Carl's drug of choice was alcohol in quantities that could be considered pretty much insane. He lived a self-described rock-and-roll lifestyle. He went out every night, got wasted and was lucky to make it all the way home before passing out. Toward the end of his 20s, he looked at his own body and discovered that he was fat, bloated and felt awful most of the time.

Somewhere deep within his evolutionary programming a bell went off. He recognized that he stood at a personal crossroads. It was time to make a decision: clean himself up and balance his rock and roll dreams with a healthier lifestyle or die like Elvis, slumped over a toilet. *The Drunk Diet* is Carl's story of getting healthy—not necessarily clean—along with the diet and exercise plan he developed along the way.

> **Fact:** We have a friend in New York City who played in a dozen different bands and, at one point, even opened for Nirvana. In her youth, she partied every

night imitating the live-fast lifestyle of her rock heroes. These days, she is rapidly running out of friends. One by one, all of the people she performed and partied with overdosed and/or committed suicide. Like Carl, she cleaned up her act just in time. She managed to get out with few long-term negative consequences and a thousand great stories.

We don't share these dramatic turnarounds. We never rocked all that hard. Andrea tended bar for a while, but never fully committed to the lifestyle. Steven is a musician, but the ukulele just doesn't lend itself to being smashed on stage. All we can say is that if our friend and Lüc Carl ever start a rock-and-roll Survivors Club, we hope we're invited along to listen to them compare war stories.

The Drunk Diet is so intertwined with Carl's personal story that it can be difficult at times to ferret out actual advice. Like us, Carl dramatically limits sugar. His acceptable food list differs from ours in that he allows bread, pasta and sandwich wraps as long as they are of the whole-grain variety. He makes no effort to hide his disdain for diets like Drink Your Carbs that eliminate these foods: "This no-carbs craze is a bunch of bullshit."

Carl also avoids salt and high-fat foods, including red meat and egg yolks. By contrast, we pretty much live on red meat and eggs, yolks included. And our enthusiasm for salt can only be compared to a deer loving up a saltlick.

Fact: Our favorite rule in *The Drunk Diet* is that Carl will not purchase any foods containing ingredients he can't pronounce. This effectively removes all processed food. Everyone should adopt this, unless, of course,

> you're a food scientist who knows how to pronounce these words. In that case you should avoid purchasing foods that include ingredients that Carl can't pronounce.

The most important component of *The Drunk Diet* is that Carl dramatically limits his portion sizes. If he makes a pot of chili or a big bowl of whole-wheat pasta, he immediately divides it into separate containers and puts them away in his fridge. What most people would eat in a single serving he spreads over several days. This is a very different approach than we take with our Food List, but anyone who has tried Weight Watchers, Jenny Craig or any one of the dozens of other diets based on reducing portion sizes can attest to the fact that this methodology works.

> **The Drunk Diet Fashion Advice:** Running in "spandex pants [is] much more comfortable, and way more Rock 'N' Roll."

Carl's approved list of alcohol is as small as his pasta dinner in a Tupperware marked "Thursday" in his fridge. Carl drinks little, if any, beer. He orders wine only occasionally. He avoids mixers for the same reasons we do. His go-to cocktail is vodka, soda and lime. And he insists that bartenders mix it weak so that he can down them all night without getting too sloppy. This has to be the most difficult part of his routine. Carl is, among other things, a bartender. Bartenders don't mix weak drinks for other bartenders. He doesn't say how he pulls off his half-portion vodka sodas, but our guess is that he has to beg.

Like Drink Your Carbs, *The Drunk Diet* demands exercise. And once again, Carl takes a very personal approach to his recommendations. Carl walks through his own journey from couch potato to marathon runner in order to provide a step-by-step exercise plan. He focuses on running because he clearly enjoys it. In his own words: "going on a run feels (almost) as good as getting laid."

We've had great runs in beautiful locations but we have yet to feel that level of euphoria. Carl does include music recommendations for running; at some point we may try running to his mix to see if that helps.

Fact: We'll be honest. We can't evaluate Carl's music list because we know nothing about heavy metal. Andrea grew up in a hippy household listening to classic 60s and 70s rock. Steven was a fan of punk and new wave, which, for reasons he can no longer recount, meant that he refused to listen to metal. To be fair, his friends who listened to metal felt the same way about his music.

In order to gain perspective on Carl's music recommendations, we called our friend Josh who happens to be a heavy metal bassist. He's not famous. These days, most of his work is done in the form of duets with his 11-year-old son who's learning guitar. We shared Carl's playlist, but failed to mention that Carl prefers listening to whole albums. Based on our friend's response, that information appears to have been important:

"This list covers a somewhat random and very wide range of metal styles from high pitched, screamy pop metal (Iron Maiden, Motley Crue) to borderline classic rock metal (early Van Halen, AC/DC, Motorhead) to fast and furious hardcore metal (Slayer, early Metallica). These bands are far apart in terms of their metal styles. I mention this because if you put a playlist together with all of them it would be a pretty rough transition

> from one song to the next. Kind of like watching *Jurassic Park* and then switching straight over to *Barney.* Both feature dinosaurs but are otherwise very different pieces of entertainment."

We have no doubt that *The Drunk Diet* works. If you follow Carl's recommendations you'll be eating small portions and exercising daily. You'll be drinking far fewer calories than are allowed on Drink Your Carbs. According to Carl, "diet books are really a whole bunch of crap written by a whole bunch of assholes who think they know more about your body than you do."

We respectfully disagree. *The Drunk Diet* contains great information for the committed drinker who also wants to lose weight. It's a very different path from Drink Your Carbs, but if your plans include throwing an amplifier off a fourth story balcony this book contains a lot of sound advice that Drink Your Carbs lacks.

Where to Find These Books

If you want to read *Letter on Corpulence, Addressed to the Public*, it is out of copyright and available online for free at Archive.org.

If you are interested in checking out either of the other two books, *The Drinking Man's Diet* and *The Drunk Diet,* are both still in print. They can be purchased from Amazon, but we encourage you to instead order them through a local bookstore. We love Amazon, but two small bookstores recently closed within half a mile of our house. We don't want to live in a world without small, independent booksellers.

We like browsing through stacks of books. We love the smell of paper. There are small mysteries and political statement that vanish when books are listed in a database; for example, are the works of Richard Dawkins shelved under Science or Religion? We even enjoy the creepy men who sit for hours on worn-out couches pretending to read Foucault in the mistaken assumption that it will make them more attractive to the opposite sex. So please, let Amazon ship you toilet paper, but if you want a copy of either of these books, order them through a local store.

Thirty Two

Recipes

Flip through any popular diet book and you will notice that they all have one thing in common: the explanation of the diet is short enough to be written on the back of a matchbook cover. "Eat Less." "No Carbs." "Exercise More." The vast majority of the bulk comes from Food lists that most people skim past and recipes no one will ever attempt.

For the record, authors of diets do not expect you to prepare any of their recipes. If you don't believe us, try a random recipe from a random diet book. More likely than not, you will find it unworkable. They are frequently missing key ingredients and directions. The measurements are often inaccurate. The final results typically range from bland to inedible. These recipes also occasionally contradict the advice dispensed in the diet.

> **Fact:** Rob Wolf's bestselling diet book, *The Paleo Solution*, forbids all legumes including peanuts, peas and all varieties beans. According to Wolf, legumes are "[g]ut irritating . . . antinutrients."[1]
>
> It should come as no surprise that *The Paleo Solution* includes a recipe for roasted green beans.[2]
>
> Nearly every diet book we have read reflects this same attitude: recipes are so inconsequential they don't warrant proofreading.

We are taking a very different approach. Instead of including 50 recipes no one will ever attempt, we have included eight recipes that we make all the time. These are some of our favorite foods. Moreover, we tested all of these recipes on strangers. We have been assured that they are as easy-to-follow as they are healthy and delicious.

Three Awesome Salad Dressings

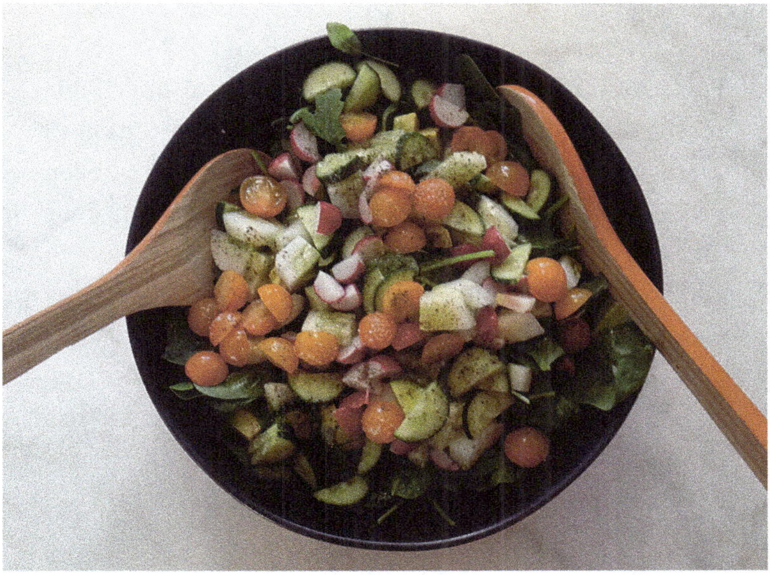

"If you want dessert, you're going to have to eat that salad." Growing up in Steven's house, a plate of leafy greens was viewed as a punishment. Each of the kids was required to consume at least a few pieces of iceberg lettuce drowning in bottled ranch dressing. Steven, in particular, responded to it as though he was being asked to eat a live cockroach.

Contrast this with Andrea's house. There was no iceberg lettuce or store-bought dressing sweetened with high-fructose corn syrup and pumped full of chemicals to increase the shelf life. Her family assembled salads of fresh romaine, tomatoes, cucumbers, carrots and other vegetables served lightly dressed in a homemade dressing.

Throughout the long Colorado summers, Andrea and her siblings would pick fresh greens and vegetables from their garden and then fight over who got to wash and cut them. The downside of all of this "kitchen help" was that someone was invariably served a slug.

> **Fact:** Assuming each person at Andrea's dinner table received an equal portion of salad, the distribution of garden mollusks throughout the family should've been random. This was not the case. More often than not—and Steven interviewed several family members to confirm this—the slug went to Andrea's younger sister Cassandra.
>
> Andrea argues that this was a naturally occurring statistical anomaly. Steven is not convinced. At the risk of sounding paranoid, when Steven looks at the grassy knoll he sees shadows of Andrea's older brother.

A bowl of lettuce is just a bowl of lettuce. It takes dressing to make a great salad. Steven's parents knew this and hoped that the food scientists at Kraft could fill that void. As we mentioned, Andrea's family made fresh dressing every night.

After all those years of practice, all of Andrea's siblings hold the equivalent of a PhD in salad dressings. They exchange tips and recipes every time they cook together. If competitive salad making were a sport, they would dominate it like the Manning brothers.

Here are three of Andrea's best vinaigrettes. Paired with fresh greens, any one of these dressings will yield perfection. (Obviously, the slugs are optional.)

Basic Balsamic Vinaigrette

Ingredients

1 medium shallot (yielding approximately 2 tbsp.)
1 small clove of garlic (optional)
2 tsp. smooth Dijon mustard
4 tbsp. balsamic vinegar (This will impact the taste of the dressing more than anything else. A sweet balsamic = sweet dressing. More acidic = stronger, more tart dressing. It's impossible to own too many balsamic vinegars. Experiment with different ones to find your favorite.)
8 tbsp. extra virgin olive oil (Feel free to add more if you like an oilier dressing. Less if you like more vinegar. Our ideal ratio is 2:1 balsamic to oil.)
1 tsp. salt
Black pepper to taste

Method

Thoroughly chop the shallot and garlic and place in a medium bowl. Add the balsamic and allow the mixture to sit for five to 10 minutes. Add the mustard. Add the salt. Mix well. It's important to add the salt at this phase because salt does not dissolve easily in oil. Once the oil is added, the salt tends to remain in the liquid like tiny grains of sand.

Slowly drizzle in olive oil while whisking. The dressing should thicken quite a bit. (The technical term is "emulsify," but most people have not seen that word since they last studied for the SAT.)

Fact: Sometimes you have to pull out a vibrator to finish having sex. (Yeah, we said it.) Similarly, sometimes you need to bring in heavy machinery to get

> dressing to emulsify. If you are struggling to thicken your dressing, use a hand blender or do the final mixing in a food processor or blender.

Add pepper to taste. Let the dressing rest for at least 10 minutes before using; this allows the flavors to combine. Re-whisk the dressing just before pouring it on to the salad.

This recipe makes more than enough for a few salads. Feel free to make it in advance, as the dressing will keep in the refrigerator for a week or more.

Champagne Vinaigrette

Ingredients

1 small clove of garlic
½ tsp. smooth Dijon mustard
2 tbsp. champagne vinegar
4 tbsp. extra virgin olive oil (Again, feel free to add more if you like an oilier dressing. Less if you like more vinegar.)
½ tsp. salt

Method

Mince the garlic and combine it with the vinegar, mustard and salt in a bowl. As with the Balsamic Dressing, mix well and then allow the mixture to rest for five to 10 minutes.

Slowly drizzle in olive oil while whisking. The dressing should thicken. Let the dressing sit for at least 10 minutes in order to unify the flavors. Re-whisk the dressing before pouring it onto the salad.

The recipe yields enough for one large salad. The dressing will keep for a week or more in the refrigerator.

Variations on the Above

- Substitute mustard with a mixture of lemon juice, orange juice or lime juice along with the champagne vinegar for light citrus component. Without mustard, the dressing will not thicken as much. (This variation is admittedly vague, but it's by design. It has to be done to taste. But here is our favorite version: Lose the mustard and use ½ orange juice and ½ champagne vinegar. This version of the dressing goes unbelievably well with duck.)
- Any light, tangy vinegar will work in place of the champagne vinegar. Examples include white sherry, white wine and light or white balsamic vinegars. Rice vinegar will also work, and it

gives the dressing a distinctly Asian flair. (To make the flavor even more Asian, add a few drops of sesame oil and ¼ tsp. chopped ginger.)

- Add finely chopped herbs (fresh tarragon, thyme, sage, basil and parley are all excellent options) to make your vinaigrette more aromatic. This is particularly good in the summer if you, like us, have fresh herbs growing in your garden.

Lemon Olive Oil Dressing

This is our favorite dressing for arugula and other bitter or peppery greens. As an added bonus, it pairs far better with wine than either of the two previous dressings. Vinegars tend to fight with wine. This dressing does not. If you want to channel your inner sommelier and match your salad course to a glass of wine, this is definitely the way to go.

Ingredients

2 tbsp. lemon juice (3 tbsp. Meyer lemon juice if you can get Meyer lemons.)
4 tbsp. extra virgin olive oil
½ tsp. salt

Method

Add the salt to lemon juice. Mix until the salt dissolves.

Slowly drizzle oil into the lemon juice while whisking vigorously. The dressing should thicken and change color to a light, milky yellow. Let the dressing rest for 10 minutes and re-whisk it just before pouring it onto the salad.

This recipe yields enough for one large salad. Leftovers will keep in the refrigerator for two to three days, but this dressing is best served immediately.

> **Note:** All these dressings are relatively low in salt. We tend to be conservative when it comes to salting food. You can always add more to your salad, but it's impossible to take salt away.

Raw Kale Salad

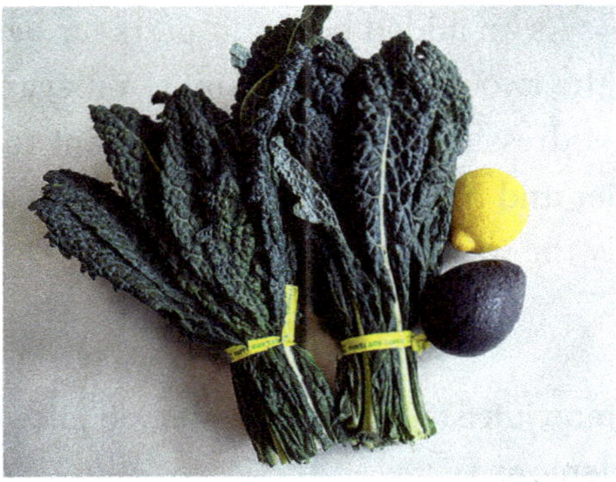

Before dating Andrea, Steven lived on ramen noodles and Taco Bell. Friends can vouch for the fact that he would occasionally eat at Taco Bell twice in the same day. He maintained a Costco membership solely to purchase ramen by the carload. On the rare occasions he craved vegetables, he headed over to a buck-a-scoop Chinese place for a version of beef with broccoli that likely contained as much MSG as broccoli.

Steven did not even know that kale was edible. He had never actually seen anyone eat it. He thought it was only used to garnish salad bars. He avoided salad bars at all cost. To Steven's pre-Andrea way of thinking, salad was for losers.

Andrea taught Steven that kale is delicious. The first time she cooked it was an epiphany. It not only tasted great, it made Steven feel good as well. He had no idea that food could make him feel anything more than full, that it could leave him physically nourished, happy and energetic. When your favorite foods are Nachos Bell Grande and Cup-O-Noodle, the nourishing quality of food is not an observation you have an opportunity to make.

Fact: There are a few tricks, but prepared properly, the garnish can be the tastiest thing on the salad bar.

Raw Kale Salad

Ingredients

2 to 3 heads of dino (or lacinato) kale. (Smaller leaves are better for salad. We recommend cooking larger kale, but when you come across bunches with small leaves, this recipe is the way to go.)

1 ripe avocado

2 tbsp. champagne vinegar

4 ½ tbsp. extra virgin olive oil (more if you prefer less vinegary salad dressing.)

2 tbsp. lemon juice

1 tsp. Salt

Pepper

Method

Wash and de-stem the kale. There are many ways to remove the stems. Andrea's preferred method involves grasping a leaf by the thickest part of the stem and wrapping her other hand tightly around the bottom of the leaf. She then pulls both hands apart in a motion that could best be described as conspicuously sexual. If you do this correctly, one hand will end up holding a naked stem and the other a handful of de-stemed kale.

Steven uses a more technical method. He carefully tears each leaf from the stem in perfect, unbroken strips. Both work. A knife works as well. You can leave in the stem at the top of the leaf from the point where it's less than 2mm thick.

Tear the prepared kale into salad sized bites and toss it into a salad bowl.

Add 1 tbsp. of the lemon juice and 1 tsp. of kosher salt. (Regular salt will work, just use a bit less as kosher salt is slightly less salty.)

Massage the kale. Squeeze and crunch the kale with your

hands. Attack your kale like a kid kneading a brand new canister of Play-Doh. The kale will gradually change color to a darker green. It takes a few minutes, but the color will change.

When the kale is uniform dark green, it's time for another massage, this time with ¼ of a ripe avocado. Once again, the goal is to mash the avocado until it coats the kale like a dressing. Let the avocado/kale mixture sit at room temperature for about 10 minutes. (The lemon will keep the avocado from turning brown. Also, the acidity in the lemon does to the kale what lime juice does to ceviche; it creates a chemical change similar to cooking.)

While you're waiting, this is an excellent time to prepare the dressing.

Mix the following in a bowl and whisk it until it thickens:

2 tbsp. champagne vinegar
4 ½ tbsp. olive oil
1 tbsp. lemon juice

Dress the kale with 2–3 tbsp. of the dressing. (We tend to prefer lighter dressing, but this is a preference you are welcome to override.) Add a little more salt and the pepper to taste.

Garnish with avocado slices.

Toasted pine nuts and/or roasted almonds also make great additions.

Serve immediately.

On rare occasions, we see kale salad on a restaurant menu. We always order it and we're usually disappointed. Most restaurants use sickly sweet dressings to cover kale's natural bitterness rather than massage the bitterness out. Massaging kale takes time, but if you try this recipe we think you'll agree it yields superior results.

Fact: It has been nearly 10 years since Steven last ate Taco Bell. He has had ramen more recently, but only because we recently visited Japan and toured the Ramen Museum in Yokohama. For those who are wondering, fresh Japanese ramen has about as much in common with Cup-O-Noodles as a can of FourLoko has in common with a proper pint of British ale.

The Burger Salad

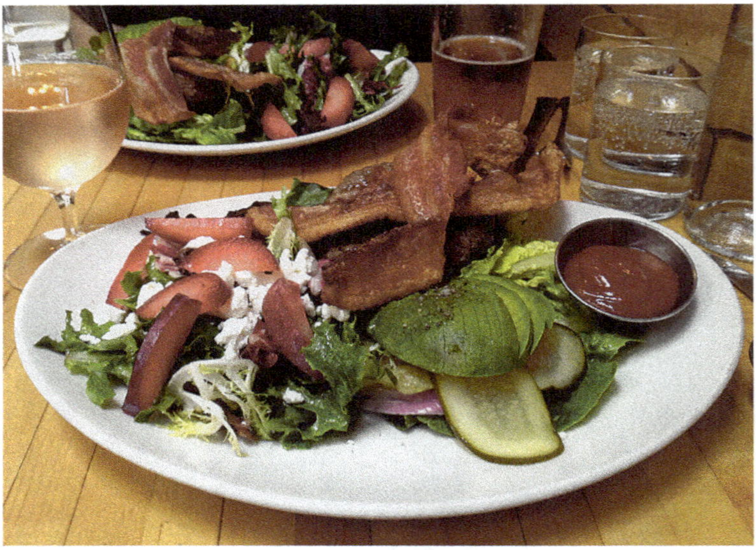

Fact: Ronald McDonald systematically destroyed lunch much in the same way John Wayne Gacy destroyed the wholesome image of clowns. (Technically, the perpetrator was McDonald's founder Ray Kroc, but we prefer to blame Ronald.)

As long as we are slandering cartoon spokesmen, we may as well share our theory that Jabba the Hutt is just Grimace after too many years of eating Happy Meals.

In 1955, McDonald's introduced the restaurant kitchen to an auto plant assembly line. The theory was that "fast and cheap" would trump "good," "fresh," and "healthy." History tells us that McDonald's was 100 percent correct. The new standard spread like meth through a rural high school or, if you prefer, like herpes through a university drama club.

Even upscale restaurants, though they are loath to admit it, have been influenced by McDonald's. Those who still serve lunch have been forced to dumb down their offerings. In order to increase service speed and decrease price, lunch menus tend to rely on simple starches. Truffled mac and cheese may sound fancy, but it is super cheap to make and shows no ill effects from spending all day in a steam drawer. In other words, it has all the same advantages as a Filet-O-Fish sandwich.

After years of cobbling together lunch from a side salad and a couple of non-fried appetizers, we finally happened upon our perfect order: the Burger Salad.

In its simplest form, the Burger Salad is a hamburger, sitting on a bed of lettuce. No bun and definitely no fries. But it can be so much more. Crisp bacon, avocado, grilled onions and even a fried egg all can make the dish as satisfying as the best burgers in the world. The Burger Salad always feels like a treat. It really does feel like cheating on your diet even though it most certainly is not. The only problem is that while it's easy to find a generic Burger Salad, it's difficult to track down a really good one.

Here is our advice for ordering the perfect Burger Salad at a restaurant. First, start by ordering a burger, not a salad. We aren't sure why, but our experience is that adding a burger to a salad seems to confuse and upset wait staff whereas a burger with an added salad makes more sense.

Next, request no bun and substitute a salad for the fries. That's the Burger Salad in its most basic form. We always ask for extra greens (in other words, we want a BIG salad.) We also specify the dressing in order to avoid having the salad smothered in something sickly sweet.

Now, on to the burger. First and foremost, say yes to add-ons. The more stuff you pile on top the better. If you're into cheese, this is an excellent time to get some. Remember that you're eating this with a knife and fork, if it sounds messy, all the better. Finally, be sure to order any and all available condiments, provided they don't contain sugar. Andrea always gets mayo or aioli. Steven is all about mustard.

> **Fact:** The search for the perfect Burger Salad is a bit like the quest for the Holy Grail. When you find it, you will know. As you search, prepare yourself for some serious disappointments, but as the old cliché goes, you have to kiss a lot of frogs in order to find a prince. Coincidentally, that same philosophy also explains how the entire university drama club came to contract herpes.

Our Secrets for Crafting Perfect Burger Salad at Home

If you want to create amazing burger salads at home, the first thing you should do is ignore all cooking advice from government bureaucrats. According to the USDA, the perfectly grilled hamburger should be cooked to an internal temperature of at least 160°F. Have you tried a 160 degree burger? We have. Andrea described the taste as, "like bobbing for apples in a bag of charcoal."

Allow us to quote the USDA website: "Many people assume that if a hamburger is brown in the middle, it is done. However, looking at the color and texture of food is not enough—you have to use a food thermometer to be sure! According to USDA research, **one out of every four** hamburgers turns brown before it reaches a safe internal temperature." (Emphasis and exclamation mark theirs.)[1]

> **Fact:** Unless you grew up in a vegetarian household, you undoubtedly have attended or even hosted a family barbeque where the burgers cooked for so long

that they had more crunch than the potato chips. The important thing to appreciate is that even these burgers may have been undercooked by USDA standards.

In Steven's family the protocol for dealing with awkward events, such as inedible food served up by an oblivious uncle, was to lie. Take a small bite, smile, nod appreciatively and pretend to enjoy it. Then sneak away and feed the rest to the dog.

Andrea's family is far more honest. If they don't like a Christmas present they look the giver straight in the eyes and ask for the gift receipt. Serve one of her brothers a burned burger and you're likely to hear, "So this is what black lung tastes like."

To be clear, we're not recommending you risk your life by eating meat cooked medium rare. We'll leave that to the Food Network. The Food Network's website provides a chart contrasting their preferred meat temperatures against the UDSA's. "Our rule of thumb," the network states, "is that if we know and trust where our meat comes from, we're okay sticking a fork in it before the USDA says it's done."[2]

Fact: The Food Network is run by cowards. They talk a good game, but just below their declaration that USDA warnings need not be heeded is a chart labeled, "Meat and Poultry Temperature Guide." While every other cut of meat is broken into rare, medium and well done, the chart offers only a single temperature for ground beef: 160°F.

We have watched Bobby Flay's *BBQ Addiction* on the Food Network. We have eaten in a number of Flay's restaurants. He does not practice what his

> parent company preaches. As far as we can tell, none of their stars do. In fact, if you search the Food Network website, you will find Emeril Lagasse's recipe for Steak Tartare. (It contains a warning about consuming raw eggs, but completely ignores the risks in consuming raw beef.)[3]

In summary, buns are bad, over-cooking is bad and condiments are good.

Tips for Crafting the Perfect Burger

Use the Best Meat You Can Find

There is no bun to hide the flavor of mediocre meat. The quality of the ingredients and the preparation are paramount. It's worth reminding yourself, the burger is the star here, and the quality of burger makes or breaks the meal. Forget about pre-formed, frozen hockey pucks. Stay away from meat that contains highly processed pink slime. The perfect burger cannot be made from inferior ingredients.

Find the best meat you can from a source you trust. For the best results, ask your butcher or meat counter to grind meat fresh for you. They rarely advertise this service, but they almost all offer it. It's more expensive than buying meat in shrink-wrapped packages, but you really can taste the difference.

Sirloin is the standard cut for burgers, but definitely experiment with others. A good butcher will guide you toward perfection.

Alternatively, you can find a butcher who grinds meat daily. Our current favorite source is 4505 Meats in San Francisco. They grind grass-fed, organic beef every morning and usually grind for a second time in the afternoon. We would put their meat up against any fresh grind in the country.

A good rule of thumb is to purchase ⅓ lb. ground beef per person.

Do Not Fear Fat

When it comes to burgers, fat is your friend. Lean beef (95 percent) makes for dry burgers. Do not worry about calories in the beef. Instead, do what we do: skip the bun, chips and high-fructose corn syrup (also known as ketchup). If you are still hungry, eat a second one. Two burgers eaten on salad will contain far fewer calories than a single burger accompanied by all the traditional fixings.

We prefer 80 percent to 85 percent lean beef. There is more moisture and that means more flavor. If it doesn't drip, you might as well be eating a dried out chicken breast.

Season Your Meat

In your perfect burger mix, spices are your friends; salt is your enemy. Salt acts like a mosquito, sucking all of the moisture and flavor out of the meat. Add herbs, spices, diced onion, garlic and peppers, but add salt only to the outside of the patties and do it just before grilling.

Blend in your spices as gently as possible. Kneading meat leads to dense, rubbery burgers. You goal should be to do the absolute minimum of mixing to distribute the seasoning evenly.

Total seasoning should be around 1 teaspoon per pound of meat. It's obvious but nonetheless worth stating—the teaspoon per pound rule can vary with intense ingredients. A teaspoon of finely chopped habanero pepper, for example, would be enough to render a pound of meat inedible to most of the population.

Pack Your Patties Loosely

The ads in the back of comic books for the Charles Atlas Dynamic-Tension bodybuilding system presented a muscle-bound man pressing the palm of his hands together as though he was trying to crush a lump of coal into a diamond. A lot of people have adopted this model for patty forming. This is a terrible idea.

A good burger will have air pockets where the fat has dripped away. Compressing the meat prevents these air pockets from forming and gives the resulting burgers a meatball-like density.

Be firm with the meat. Don't leave it so loose that it falls apart on the grill, but don't make it a strength-training exercise. You want air pockets to form.

The leaner your meat, the looser your burgers should be packed. For example, buffalo burgers—which are nearly as lean as chicken breasts—should be right on the edge of breaking apart. Since there is not enough fat to drip out and form air pockets, these hollows must be produced as part of the patties. The only way to accomplish this is to pack the meat as loosely as possible.

One last thing: don't press on your burgers with a spatula. It adds unwanted density while squeezing out flavor.

Let Your Meat Rest

For years, we assumed that it was normal to take a bite of a burger and watch all of the juices rush out like a waterfall on the plate. It turns out that resting the meat after cooking it can minimize this phenomenon.

Use the rule of fives. Pull the burgers five degrees before they reach your desired temperature. Cover them with foil and allow them to rest for five full minutes. The meat will continue cooking to the desired temperature. It will also reabsorb all of the moisture, resulting in perfectly juicy burgers.

You can quickly sear the burgers on the grill after the rest if the temperature has dropped too much. Otherwise, simply serve and enjoy.

Make a Salad Worthy of Your Burger

Use any of our Salad Dressing recipes. All of these will compliment your burger. The only additional advice we can offer is always use the freshest ingredients you can find and make twice as much salad as you think that you will need. It really is that good.

The Risk-Taker's, Adrenaline Junkie Guide to Burger Temperature

Rare: 125°
Medium-Rare: 130°
Medium: 140°
Medium-Well: 150°
Well-Done (USDA rare): 160°

We recommend using a thermometer for cooking burgers, but our reason is the opposite of that advocated by the USDA. The primary purpose of a thermometer is to ensure meat is not overcooked. Certainly, it will provide feedback if the center of your burger is still raw, but the vast majority of the time temperature readings are all about determining when to pull the meat to allow it to rest.

> **Fact:** There is some disagreement over how to construct the final burger salad. Some people place the burger onto a bed of salad and then bury it in toppings. It looks nice, but the heat from the burger tends to wilt the lettuce. We serve our burgers and toppings next to the salad and then combine all of the ingredients bite by bite. Either way, we are sure you will love the results.

Chicken alla Milanese

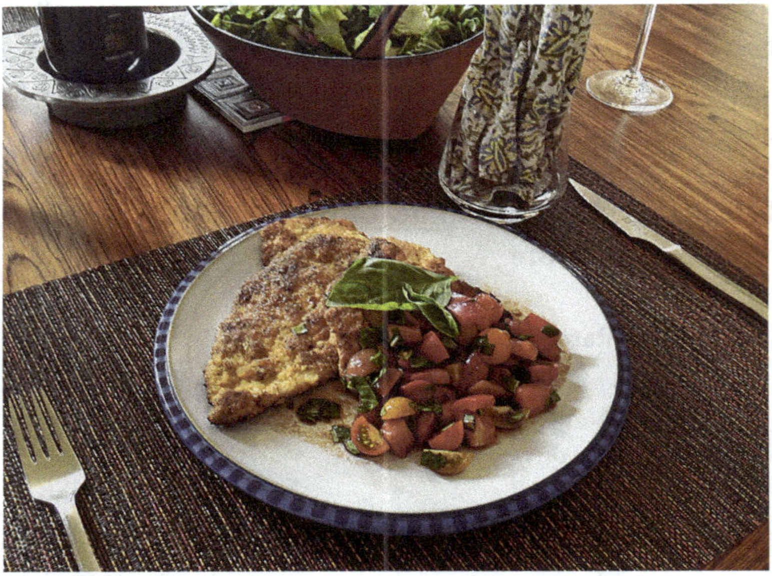

If Colonel Sanders ever embraces Drink Your Carbs, this will be the replacement for the Original Recipe™.

This is highly unlikely since the Colonel died in 1980, but it is not impossible. All it requires is a monumental shift in KFC corporate philosophy and Tupac's special effects team.

Fact: No individual KFC executive knows the complete Original Recipe. The company divides knowledge of the 11 herbs and spices among three people who, we assume, are never allowed to book seats on the same flight. This means that somewhere in the organization is a loyal executive who spent years climbing the chain of command to learn that he or she is trusted only as far as "salt, pepper and MSG."

We hold a very different attitude. When our parents admonished us to share our toys, we took it seriously. This is our Secret Recipe in its entirety. Future billion dollar chicken franchise be damned.

For anyone who has never tasted Chicken *alla Milanese*, the traditional Italian preparation is a chicken breast that is pounded thin before being breaded and deep-fried. It's sauced with fresh tomatoes, basil and balsamic vinegar. The Drink Your Carbs version looks and tastes exactly like Chicken *alla Milanese*, but it's low-carb and never goes near a fryer. It also happens to be gluten and dairy-free.

Chicken alla Milanese

Ingredients

6 boneless, skinless chicken breast halves with tenderloins removed. (For anyone unfamiliar with the tenderloin, it's the finger-sized piece of chicken meat attached to the underside of the breast. We remove the tenderloin because the dish looks better without it. We save these in a Ziploc and use them the next day in a stir-fry or any other recipe that calls for small strips of chicken.)
1 ¼ cups finely ground and blanched almond flour (This is sometimes called "almond meal." Our favorite is Benefit Your Life organic almond flour, but any brand will work.)
2 tsp. garlic powder
1 tbsp. salt
1 tbsp. ground black pepper
2 eggs, beaten
3 cups coarsely chopped (½ inch squares) fresh tomatoes. (Early Girls are our favorite, but cherry tomatoes—Sweet 100s or Golden—work just as well.)
1 tbsp. extra virgin olive oil
¼ cup chopped fresh basil, plus 4 whole basil leaves for garnish
3 tbsp. balsamic vinegar
Salt and freshly ground black pepper to taste
Additional oil for searing

Method

1. Preheat oven to 400°. Lightly oil a large baking sheet. (We prefer to use coconut oil for this, but you can use any oil that can handle high heat.) Place the oiled baking sheet in the oven to heat up;

2. In a large bowl, mix the tomatoes and chopped basil together and add the olive oil, balsamic, salt and freshly ground pepper. Allow the mixture to rest for at least 10 minutes before serving;
3. Using a chef's mallet, frying pan or rolling pin (choose your weapon from anything that will flatten the chicken), gently beat the chicken breast halves between two sheets of plastic wrap or parchment paper. The goal is to flatten them to around ¼ inch thick. Try not to beat on them too hard or you risk spraying raw chicken across your kitchen. If you've ever seen the comedian Gallagher smash a watermelon you know exactly the technique you want to avoid;
4. Mix the almond flour, garlic powder, salt and pepper in a bowl. A wire whisk works well for this. Be sure to break up any chunks in the almond flour so the resulting mix is smooth;
5. Pre-heat about 1 tsp. of olive or coconut oil on medium high heat in a large non-stick frying pan. You want the chicken to sizzle when you put it in, but not burn;
6. Working with one piece of chicken at a time, dip the chicken into the egg and then dredge it through the almond flour mixture. If it's done correctly, a light coating of the flour should now cover the entire piece of chicken. Sear each side of the chicken for approximately one minute until it becomes crispy and golden brown. Use tongs to gently transfer each piece of chicken onto the pan in the oven, being careful not to knock off the lovely coating. Repeat this process until all of your chicken is done and resting in the oven;
7. If the oil gets too hot (immediately blackens the chicken breast) or turns to a dark brown, dump the oil out, wipe the pan clean and start with fresh, pre-heated oil for the next piece of chicken;

8. Allow the chicken to sit in the oven for 2–3 minutes after the last breast has been seared. This ensures both the almond flour and chicken are fully cooked;
9. Serve the chicken breast topped with ½ cup of the cold tomato mixture. Garnish with a whole basil leaf. Serve immediately.

You may have noticed that we include far fewer than 11 herbs and spices. Simply add more spices if you feel the need to crank your blend up to 11. But do beware of the Curse of the Colonel.

We know this sounds crazy, but the Curse of the Colonel is real. In 1985, the Hanshin Tigers of Kansai Japan won the Japan Series, the Japanese equivalent to the World Series. Fans went wild and swarmed into the street. For reasons that we will never understand, in the midst of their euphoric celebrations, fans stole a fiberglass statue of Colonel Sanders from an Osaka KFC franchise and threw it, with great ceremony, off a bridge into a river.

The very next season, the Hanshin Tigers began an extended losing streak and the Curse of the Colonel, or *Kāneru Sandāsu no Noroi*, was born. We would be tempted to laugh at the superstitiousness of Japanese baseball fans, but the truth is that Hanshin's curse is no different from the Chicago Cubs' Curse of the Billy Goat or the Red Sox Curse of the Bambino.

In a 2005 interview with the Taipei Times, then President of KFC, Gregg Dedrick, ominously warned "anyone divulging [the secret blend] might incur the curse of the Colonel."[1] If you're superstitious and a baseball fan, the last thing you want to do is to happen upon the secret blend accidentally. If this were to occur, the simple act of innocently sharing your version with a friend would unleash the Colonel's fury. Superstitious baseball fans should play it safe and stop adding herbs and spices when they reach 10.

Easy Green Sauce

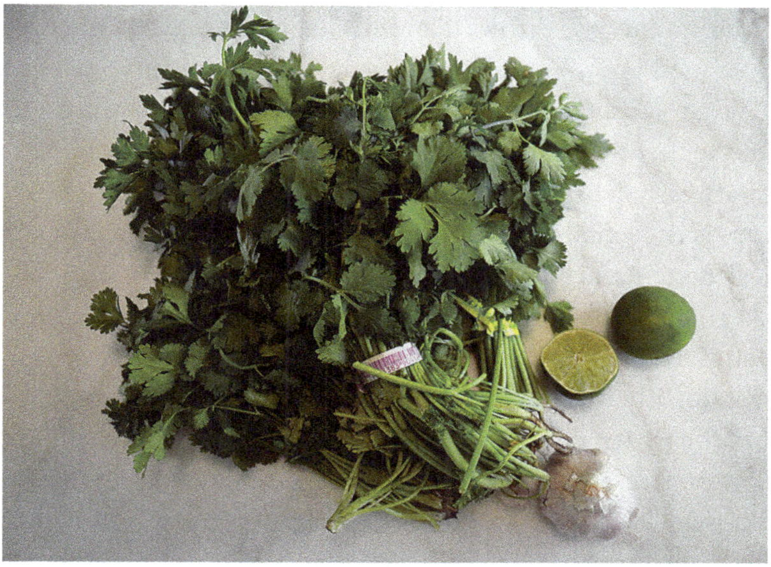

There is nothing that cannot be improved by the addition of either chocolate or bacon. Before we discovered Drink Your Carbs, this was our culinary philosophy. Bacon is still a mainstay, but chocolate is now a rare occurrence.

These days we have a new philosophy: everything is better with either bacon or Green Sauce. The truth is, if you add our Green Sauce, bacon is unnecessary. Green Sauce really is that good. We have yet to discover any meat or vegetable that is not improved by it.

The original recipe, before we added our own modifications, came from our dear friend and CrossFit trainer, Monica Ward. Monica is the reason we are both able to do pull-ups and execute beautiful overhead squats. More than once, she has drunk us under the table in the evening and then coached us through a nasty workout first thing the next morning. These are only a few of the reasons that Monica received the very first Drink Your Carbs Lifetime Achievement Award.

Monica's Green Sauce is a fairly traditional chimichurri. The recipe is as easy as it is tasty.

Monica simply throws handfuls of herbs, spices and garlic into a food processor. She adds olive oil and presses "start." The resulting sauce transformed an ordinary grilled flatiron steak into the best Mexican-style cut of meat we had ever tasted. We've been tweaking her original recipe ever since. The beauty of Green Sauce is its flexibility. Minor variations transform the flavor from Mexican to French to Italian to Middle Eastern.

It might just be the perfect food. Aside from the extraordinary level of flavor it adds to just about anything, Green Sauce stores exceptionally well. You can pour it into an ice cube tray and then store the frozen cubes in a Ziploc for later use. We typically keep three or four versions on hand. We'll make a huge batch and then thaw it cube by cube over the following months. There are times when our freezer would qualify us to be on an episode of *Hoarders*.

Easy Green Sauce

Ingredients

1 cup parsley leaves
1 cup cilantro leaves
1 clove garlic
½ tsp. salt
Cayenne to taste (Adding spice is optional)
2 tbsp. fresh lime juice
1 tbsp. hot water
½ cup olive oil

Method

1. Chop the garlic in a food processor until thoroughly minced. Don't be surprised if the garlic clove bounces around like a superball in a phone booth. Pulsing rather than letting the processor run wild usually settles it down enough to mince it;
2. If you have not done so already, pick the herb leaves off of the stems, wash them and dry them. This might be the most time-consuming part of the recipe, but trust us; it's well worth the effort. Stems can add an odd texture and unwanted bitterness to the sauce. This step is the main reason we like to make a lot of Green Sauce and freeze it. It might be boring and repetitive, but once you start removing stems from herbs, it's easy to keep the momentum going;
3. Add the herbs to the garlic in the food processor. Pulse the mixture until it is finely chopped. It's important to chop the herbs before adding any liquid to the food processor; otherwise, instead of being chopped, the herbs tend to swim around in a circle like clothes in a washing machine;
4. Add the lime juice, salt and cayenne (optional) to the food processor. Blend once again until the mixture becomes a smooth

paste. You do not need to get the herbs perfectly smooth. Just make sure the herbs are chopped finely;

5. Add the hot water. Blend and then let the mixture sit for a couple minutes;
6. With the food processor running, slowly add the olive oil. The green paste will transform into a light, oily sauce.

Taste for salt, lime and spice. Adjust as needed. This recipe is deliberately low sodium. We prefer to salt the underlying meats and vegetables. But feel free to adjust the salt to your taste.

Serve it over grilled meats, vegetables, sausage, etc. It works best to slather the sauce on food that is piping hot. The green sauce cooks slightly from the heat and develops an incredible fragrance. We always set a bowl of extra sauce on the table and it tends to disappear quickly.

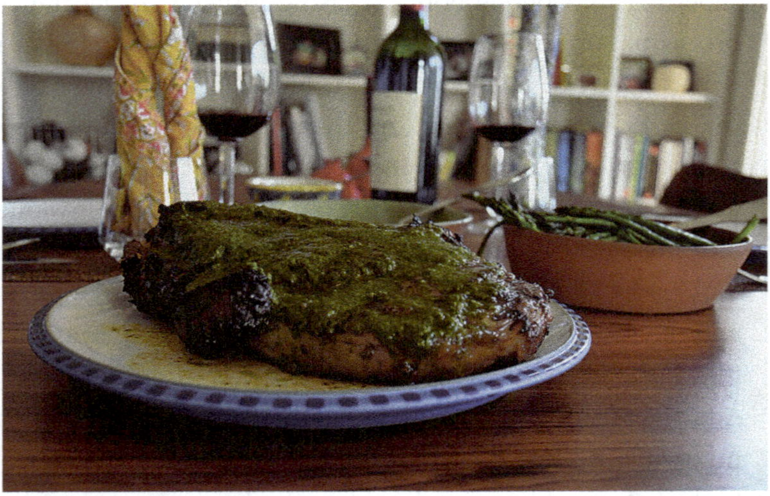

Green Sauce Variations

There are endless variations of this recipe and experimentation usually pays off. The version above is very Mexican, with lime and cilantro. However, the sauce can be made with nearly any green leafy herb and any citrus, vinegar or other acid. (The only herb exception is that we do not recommend rosemary. Rosemary tends to make the sauce unpleasantly bitter.)

Our Favorite Combinations Are

- Use sherry vinegar as a replacement for the lime and substitute the cilantro with two cups of parsley.
- Add fresh oregano to the parsley version above for an Italian flair.
- Add capers and olives to the parsley version for a briny, Mediterranean taste.
- Use lemon juice instead of lime juice to create a perfect sauce for grilled chicken breast.

The combinations are endless. Please send us an email at info@drinkyourcarbs.com if you think of something new and fun.

How to Use Frozen Cubes of Green Sauce

To unfreeze Green Sauce, it's best to remove a cube or two and let them slowly thaw to room temperature in a bowl on the kitchen counter. Don't use a microwave. You don't want the sauce to cook and even the "defrost" setting on your microwave will likely give you more heat than you want. If you're in a hurry, place the cubes in a porcelain or metal bowl, and place that bowl in another bowl of hot water. The heat will transfer and melt the cubes reasonably quickly.

Previously frozen Green Sauce can be improved by adding a touch of fresh citrus or vinegar. If you've labeled your bag of cubes (we write the date and the recipe used on the Ziploc with a permanent ink marker), simply add more of the original acidic component (lime, vinegar, lemon etc.). One teaspoon or less per cube is enough to brighten the flavor.

We also use Green Sauce cubes to add zest to all types of recipes. Anything that calls for parsley/cilantro, etc. can benefit from a cube or two thrown in during the cooking phase. Simply add the cubes and be sure that they melt completely. Then simmer the recipe you're making for at least two minutes. Cooking for longer is fine. Our two-minute recommendation is the minimum required to integrate the Green Sauce into your food.

Again, play with this. Let us know what you do. If anyone has the guts to throw a cube or two into a protein shake, we'd love to hear how it goes. That's one road we have been afraid to travel down.

Perfect Kale

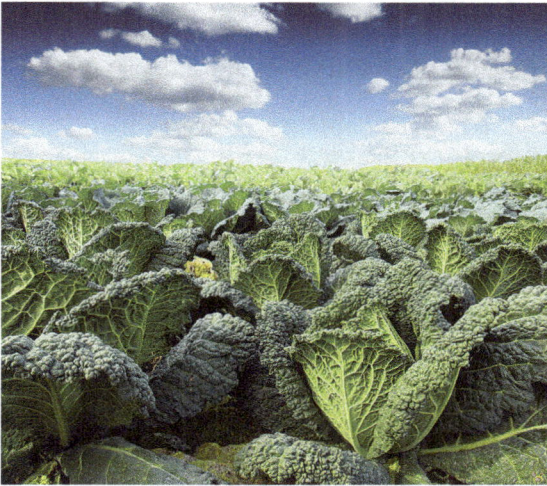

Hello. My name is Steven. I used to hate kale. Now I love it.

When did it become a virtue to never change your mind? Watch any recent election coverage and the conclusion is unavoidable. We, as a country, have decided that new information should have no impact on opinions and beliefs. If you abandon a single conviction you held in seventh grade, you're a weak-minded flip-flopper. It doesn't matter what life experiences you've had between then and now. New evidence be damned. Changing your mind for any reason betrays you as indecisive and lacking in backbone.

Go ahead and accuse me of being un-American. I have flip flopped on kale.

I used to think that kale was far too bitter. It turns that my dislike of kale had everything to do with how it was prepared. The minute I tasted Andrea's kale it became my favorite vegetable. Andrea and I are now in complete agreement that kale is the world's most perfect vegetable. It's low-calorie and high-nutrition. It's delicious. It is the perfect compliment to any Drink Your Carbs meal.

Perfect Kale

Ingredients

2 bunches dino kale (Other types of kale will work, but dino works best)

1–2 tbsp. extra virgin olive oil

1 slice of bacon, finely minced (Tip: freeze uncooked bacon. Frozen bacon minces easily)

2 cloves garlic, finely minced or crushed

¼–½ tsp. hot pepper flakes (Optional)

½ tsp. fish sauce (Optional) (Check the label before you buy a bottle of fish sauce. Some brands contain sugar)

1 tsp. salt (Use ½ tsp. if you are adding fish sauce)

Chicken stock or water for moisture

Method

Add 1–2 tbs. of salt to a large pot of water and bring to a boil.

De-stem and wash the kale (detailed de-stemming instructions can be found in our Raw Kale Salad recipe)

Submerge the kale in the boiling water and turn off the heat immediately after submerging the kale. Leave the kale in the water for two to four minutes. Cook thicker, larger-leafed kale for four minutes and smaller-leafed kale for two. If you have a variety of big and small kale, you don't have to boil the bunches separately. Majority rules—if it's mostly large leafed, go for four minutes. After boiling, drain the kale into a colander and set it aside.

Heat the olive oil on medium in a large flat-sided skillet or sauté pan. Add the bacon and cook until the fat is mostly gone. Be careful not to cook the bacon too hot. You want flavor, but not the flavor of burned bacon. Add the garlic and sauté for another 1–2 minutes. If you are adding the optional salt, hot pepper flakes or fish sauce add it when the garlic is done.

Add the kale to the saucepan. It should still be wet from the blanching process. This light moisture will steam the kale. Stir well. Reduce the heat to medium-low and cover the pan. Allow the kale to cook for two minutes, then stir it and check if it is done. The best way to tell if it is done is taste it. It often takes more than one two-minute cycle. Larger, thicker kale, usually requires multiple two-minute cycles. Smaller kale might be done the first time you check it. If the kale is not done and looks dry, add a bit of chicken stock or water (two teaspoons or so is sufficient. Don't let it get too wet). Do not add liquid if you think the kale is done. The goal is to have the kale nearly dry at the conclusion of the cooking process.

When the kale is done, remove the cover and remove the pan from heat. The kale can sit in the pan for up to 10 minutes (uncovered) while you finish the rest of your cooking.

Variations

- Chop one cup of shitake mushrooms and sauté them with the garlic until they are fairly soft. Use a bit of water, wine or chicken stock to deglaze the pan and then proceed with the recipe.
- If you prefer softer kale, add more liquid and cook it longer. Andrea prefers to use chicken stock to add moisture and flavor at the same time. Add no more than two teaspoons of stock at a time and be sure to let it cook off completely. You want the finished kale to be nearly dry. You may need to do the final steps of cooking with the lid off in order to accomplish this.
- For a sweeter variation, add ¼ cup raisins just before you allow the kale to simmer for the final two minutes with the lid on. Top with toasted pine nuts just before serving.

Easy Black Beans

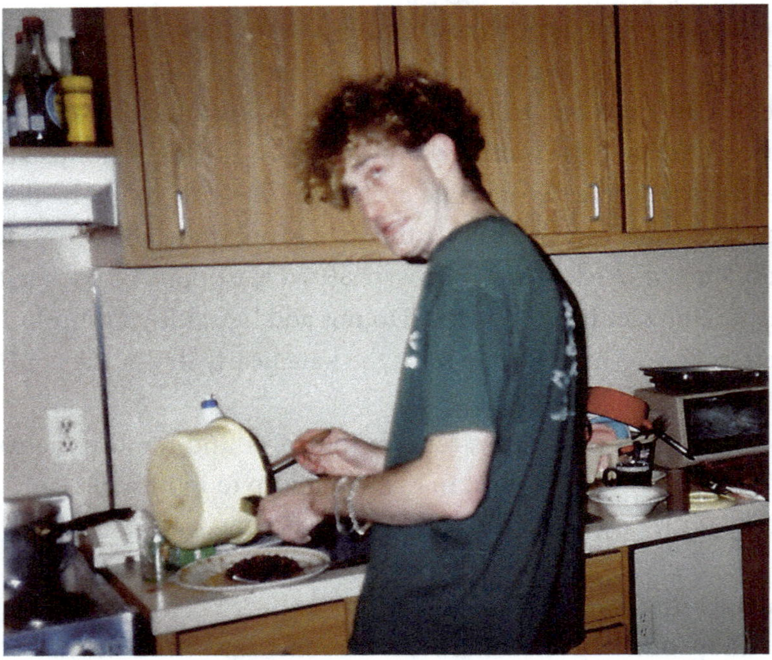

Steven cooking black beans for Andrea, 1990

Long before marrying Andrea, Steven dated a Cuban girl from Miami. It was a typical college relationship. They were madly in love within days and broken up less than six months later. The relationship had all the hallmarks of an old-fashioned melodrama. Every emotion was amplified by the inexperience and hormones of youth. After the breakup, the girl sacrificed a live chicken in order to curse Steven in a Santeria ritual. Steven probably deserved the curse; he had a tendency to crack inappropriate jokes at times when no words should be spoken. The chicken, however, was completely innocent.

It turns out that, for Steven, a cursed life is largely indistinguishable from a lucky one. Even that crazy relationship turned out to be a lucky break. Out of the wreckage, Steven managed to salvage the girl's family recipe for traditional Cuban black beans. Over the past 20 years, Andrea has taken that recipe, and, as she's prone to do, both simplified and perfected it.

The Easy Black Beans recipe violates nearly every rule we have for cooking. We believe that almost everything is better made from scratch. Stock, salad dressing, guacamole, even salsas are all superior if assembled, not bought. Our black beans, however, are decidedly not from scratch. Yet, they work brilliantly. They're as easy as microwaving popcorn. They're by far the simplest recipe we make. The results are always incredible. We think they're superior to the original recipe from which they evolved.

Easy Black Beans

Ingredients

1 can (14.5 oz.) unsalted black beans. (Read labels and try to find a brand containing only beans and water. Choose unsalted beans because the salt in canned beans varies from 100mg–700mg making the salt profile unpredictable. As a general rule, it's always best to be in charge of your own salt.)

½ can Salsa Casera (Salsa Casera is available in most grocery stores in small, 7 oz. cans) You only need half a can for the recipe. Use the rest in guacamole or throw it on eggs in the morning. Other salsas will work, but Salsa Casera is simple, contains no junk, and the results are predictably good.)

½ cup beer or chicken stock

½ cup chicken stock or water

Salt to taste (about 1 tsp.)

Method

Combine one can of black beans (including liquid), ½ can of Salsa Casera, and ½ cup beer or chicken stock in a saucepan. Bring to a low boil, then reduce the heat and simmer.

Stir frequently, until almost all the liquid is gone. Then add ½ cup chicken stock or an equivalent amount of water. Add the salt at this time as well.

Simmer again until the liquid is nearly gone. Taste once more for salt, and add more if needed. Turn off the heat and let the beans set up a bit. Serve.

It has been pointed out that these beans are no longer Cuban. Fair enough. The flavor profile in this version is far more Mexican. It is also worth mentioning that the double boil can take a while. Start the beans before you start anything else.

Drink Your Carbs Brownies

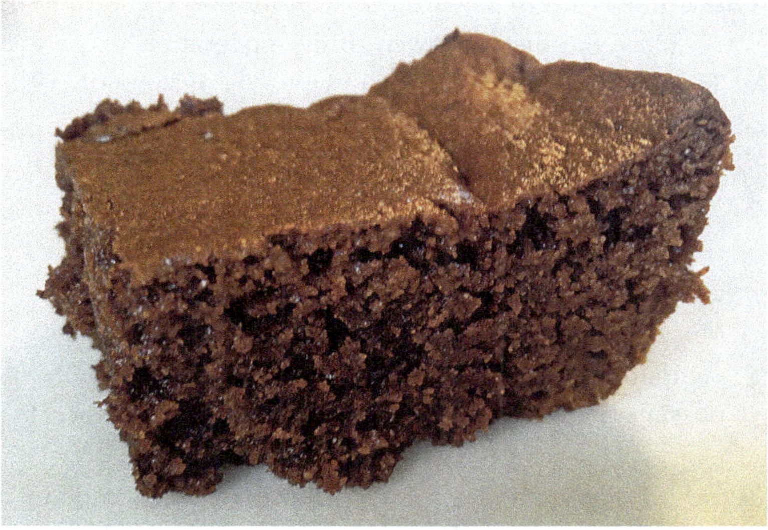

Full Disclosure: These brownies are not 100 percent Drink Your Carbs compliant. The Basic Drink Your Carbs diet eliminates both maple syrup and honey. When it comes to sweeteners, Drink Your Carbs is more restrictive than Paleo or pretty much any other diet we've seen. Our reasoning is simple. If we want to continue drinking alcohol, we have to cut calories elsewhere. Eliminating sweeteners is the easiest and most efficient way to accomplish this.

If we want something to finish a meal, our choice is invariably another glass of wine, beer or an occasional Scotch. But even we bust out this recipe for special occasions. If we plan to make dessert for a party, these are our go to choice.

Fact: Not all cheats are created equal. If you are going to treat yourself, these are the highest protein, lowest

> sugar dessert we've come across. And more importantly, they don't taste like it.

One Final Word of Warning: If you make these all the time you will blow you diet. We even think moderation is too excessive. The key here is that these brownies should remain a treat. Use them sparingly and you'll be fine; after all, on Drink Your Carbs 90% compliance is still an A.

> **Fact:** Arthur C. Clarke wrote, "Any sufficiently advanced technology is indistinguishable from magic." Most people assume he was referring to things like computers, smart phones and marital aids. It's equally possible that he was anticipating this brownie recipe.

These brownies are dairy and gluten-free. They contain no grains. They are composed almost entirely of almond butter and the chemistry behind them is as impressive as any advanced technology and/or magic that Clarke might have imagined. We have a reasonable understanding of chemistry yet we are stumped by the fact that we can mix up nut butter with a few other ingredients, shove it into the oven and pull out a tray of brownies.

> **Fact:** When we say "tray of brownies," we mean it. A while back, we served these to a friend. After taking a bite of his brownie he jumped into a full-fledged cooking intervention: "These are good, but I need to send you a real recipe."
>
> "Real recipe?" Andrea asked.
>
> "I mean a recipe that doesn't use a box." Based on color, texture and taste he assumed that the brownies came from a Betty Crocker mix.

Drink Your Carbs Brownies

Ingredients

1 (16 oz.) jar of creamy roasted almond butter.
2 eggs
1 cup of maple syrup or honey (Clover honey yields the tastiest results, if you decide to go with honey.)
1 tbsp. of vanilla extract
½ cup of cacao powder
½ tsp. of sea salt
1 tsp. of baking soda
1 cup of dark chocolate chips (We use dairy-free, non-cane sweetened and the results are awesome.)

Method

1. Grease a 9"x13" inch baking dish with coconut oil
2. In a large bowl, blend the almond butter with a hand blender until smooth. This is very important. Blending the almond butter to super smooth is key to getting the brownies to have the right texture.
3. Blend in eggs and then add the maple syrup (or honey) and the vanilla. Beat again until smooth.
4. Blend in cacao. Beat once more until smooth.
5. Blend in salt and baking soda. Beat one last time, until all of the lumps are gone and the mixture is uniform.
6. Stir in chocolate chips. It probably goes without saying, but don't use the hand blender for this step as it will reduce the chips to rubble.
7. Pour the batter into the baking dish.

Bake at 300 degrees for 45–50 minutes. All ovens vary, so around minute 40, check the brownies by inserting a toothpick into the center; the brownies are done when the toothpick comes out clean. The edge will be quite crisp. This is a good thing.

Allow the brownies to cool completely before cutting. If we can restrain ourselves, we make them the night before and leave them to cool overnight lightly covered with a towel. As strange as this sounds, they are better the second day.

Variations

- Add ½ cup of chopped walnuts or pecans.
- Skip the cacao powder and add ½ cup nuts and ½ cup raisins for an awesome Almond Butter Blondie.

Credit Where Credit Is Due: This recipe was adapted from Elana's Pantry[1] (www.elanaspantry.com) who adapted it from the Celiac Chicks[2] (www.celiacchicks.com). We definitely recommend both websites for anyone looking for grain-free recipes. One caveat: The Celiac Chicks website appears to be hosted on an old Speak & Spell. The site fails more often than it loads. Keep trying and you'll eventually get in.

Thirty Three

Cocktails

Years ago we lived next door to Dave Elger, star of the low-budget TV show, "Hot Mixology." The show's concept is simple: Community Theater meets *Leaving Las Vegas*. When Charlie Sheen embarked on his post-meltdown comedy tour a few years ago, he was stealing Dave's act.

One evening, Dave convinced us to join him on camera in the role of bar patrons. The moment a stranger dragged us into a lighted hallway and began coating us in layers of hairspray and makeup, we realized that we had made a terrible mistake. Andrea's hair was teased to Debbie Harry perfection. The layers of CoverGirl on Steven's neck and face were so thick that he felt like he was wearing a rubber Nixon mask. We saw the video the following day; our onscreen personas can best described as somewhere between a Kardashian and a rodeo clown.

Even worse than the caked on makeup or the constant waiting around during endless filming was actually having to sip the drinks and pretending to enjoy them. The theme of that week's show was "Product Placement For Absinthe." Every drink set in front of us was the cocktail equivalent of Pixy Stix. In this case, we don't blame "Hot Mixology." Absinthe is bitter. The traditional way to make it palatable is to keep adding simple syrup until it is indistinguishable from ginger ale. By those standards, the drinks were excellent. From a Drink Your Carbs perspective, however, when you drink one of these it's like your diet hitting an iceberg.

Most of these drinks contained more calories from sweeteners than liquor. There are about 100 calories in a shot of Absinthe. There are 50 calories in a tablespoon of simple syrup. We estimate that each drink contained about three to four tablespoons of simple syrup.

As far as we are concerned, this is the problem with modern cocktail culture. We cannot repeat this too many times: when it comes to cocktails, follow a simple rule: No Mixers. In most cases, losing the mixers eliminates more than half the calories. If you want to continue drinking on your diet, the no-mixer rule is key.

This does not mean that you have to drink your liquor straight. It is still possible to make excellent cocktails and adhere to the rule. To prove this, we offer a few of our favorite cocktails and a mixing guide that will allow anyone to create endless cocktails of their own. Try our recipes. Then experiment with your own. It is not difficult to mix mixer-free drinks so good that even "Hot Mixology" would approve.

Fact: Our depiction of Hot Mixology is not entirely fair. We were on the show in 2010. At the time, it was a drunken Wayne's World that aired after midnight on local cable. The show is now syndicated nationwide and appears on The Cooking Channel. It is now far more professional. That said, we imagine that the hairspray, makeup and the hours of waiting around are still a valued part of the experience.

Our portrayal of Hot Mixology might be unfair, but we strongly believe that our depiction of Dave is still dead accurate. In college, Dave worked summers as a Party Catalyst for Club Med in Mexico. His job was to get people drunk enough that they were willing to participate in activities like the poolside bikini contest. Twenty-five years later this is still, fundamentally, his job.

When Dave lived next door, he had a two-car garage so packed with liquor bottles that he had to park his car on the street. Sadly we don't have any photos of that car. It was a convertible Mercedes fully wrapped into a collage of taps, bottles, shot glasses and agave plants. It was a mobile billboard advertising, "Please officer, pull me over right now and give me a breathalyzer." (We assume Dave would pass that breathalyzer; nonetheless, his car demanded one be given.)

Dave recently opened the Hot Mixology Bar and Lounge in Denver. His cocktail program has gained rave reviews. He is now a respectable tavern owner and a leader of Denver's blossoming cocktail culture. But he cannot have changed that much. His newest ride is an old school bus that has been wrapped in pictures of bottles, liquor logos and a gigantic portrait of Dave himself, presumably in case the police are unsure who to breathalyze.

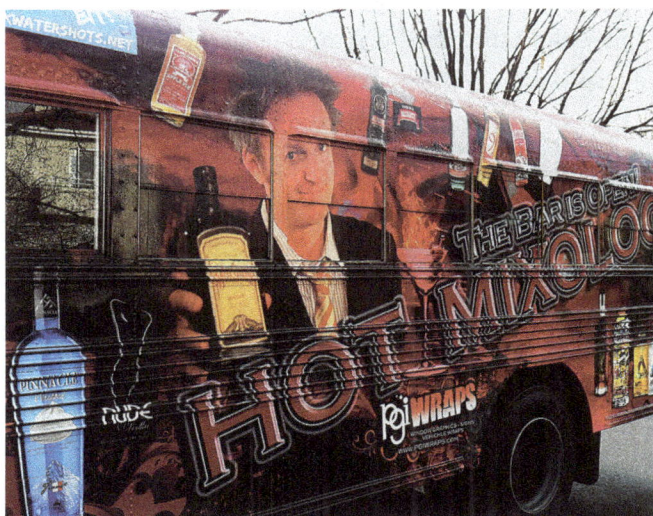

The Drink Your Carbs Margarita

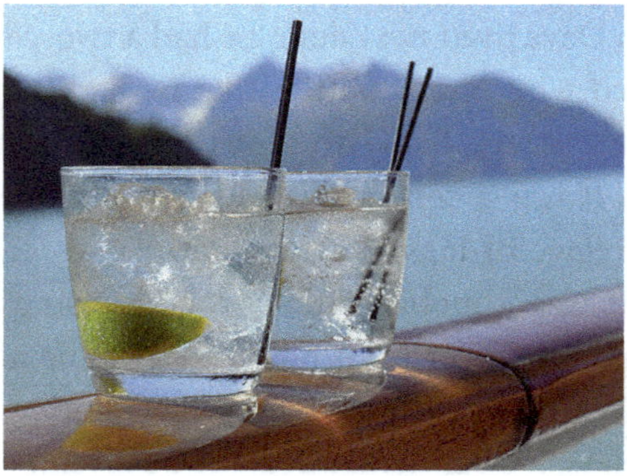

We could insist that we invented this cocktail. Everybody else does. In fact, so many people have claimed this particular recipe that we have no idea who to cite. Followers of the Paleolithic Diet refer to it as "The Paleo Margarita." Atkins, South Beach and Zone have all made claim to it under similar, "-rita" appended names. Mexico refers to it simply as the original Margarita recipe from the time before hotel bartenders sugared it up to make it more palatable to tourists.

For the sake of proper citation: The Drink Your Carbs Margarita originated somewhere between two and 10,000 years ago. It probably originated in the Americas, since the agave required to make tequila is a native plant. The most likely scenario is that the drink was invented in Mexico and we stole it without giving them credit, just like we did with Texas.

Ingredients and Method

1 oz. fresh squeezed lime juice.

1 oz. tequila. We prefer a Resposado. Feel free to experiment to find your favorite distiller/aging profile.

Fill the rest of the glass with soda water and ice.

Garnish with slices of fresh lime.

The Amaro Cocktail

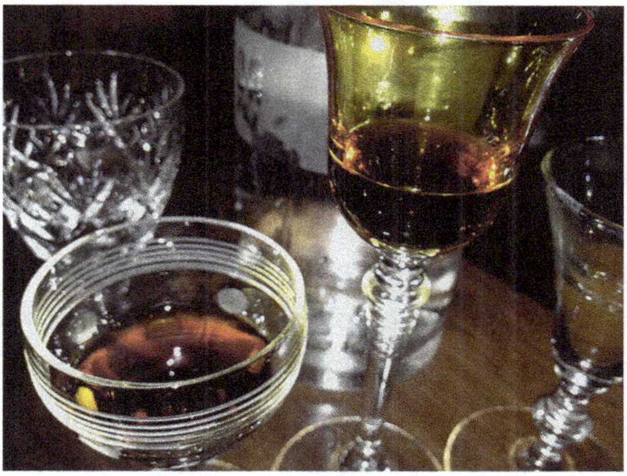

Fact: Amaro is woven into the history of Italy as deeply as pasta and Roman Catholic guilt.

The first time we tasted Amaro was in Florence, Italy more than 20 years ago. Andrea pointed to a strange looking bottle on a high shelf in a small restaurant and asked, "What is that?"

The waiter rolled his eyes, "That is for old Italian men."

Andrea didn't miss a beat. "Perfect. We'll have two served however the old men drink it."

Our drinks arrived straight up in dessert wine glasses. They were the color of long-neglected motor oil. They tasted like a mishmash of vanilla, caramel, juniper berries, peppermint and Vicks VapoRub. If we believed in past lives we might claim that we were once old Italian men because we fell instantly in love.

We later learned that Amaro is a broad category of herbal liquors made by macerating herbs in a neutral spirit. Flavors and styles vary wildly. Some are barrel aged; some are heavily sweetened. Before we order Amaro, we always ask if it is in the sweet or bitter style. If the answer is "sweet," we choose something else.

We are lucky to live in the Bay Area where Amaro is widely

available. It might be more difficult to find in other places. It is often available in large liquor stores and it can be easily ordered over the Internet (in states that allow interstate alcohol purchases). Also, we designed our recipe using the Averna brand. Averna is one of the largest Amaro producers. This should make it a little easier to track down.

Ingredients

1oz. (one shot) Averna Amaro (If you can't find Averna, any non-sweet Amaro will work. Unfortunately the only way to know if an Amaro is sweet without opening the bottle is to ask. Amaros are not marked in any way to indicate which ones are deliciously bitter and which taste like mentholated Junior Mints.)
3 oz. sparkling water
1 squeeze lime (¼ lime wedge.)
Ice

Method

Place the ice in a 6 oz. low-ball cocktail glass. Pour the Amaro over the ice. Add the soda and squeeze the lime. Drop the lime into the glass as a garnish.

Calories

An ounce of Averna contains 73 calories. A squeeze of lime is about three calories. This amounts to 19 fewer calories than in a bottle Michelob ULTRA, the second worst tasting beer-like drink in the history of brewing. If you want to taste the absolute worst, you have to track down a bottle of Zima. This is not an impossible task. Zima is no longer available in the United States, but the Coors Brewing Company still sells it in Japan where, we presume, it is used to strip auto parts.

Bartender's Guide to Mixing Unimaginative Drinks

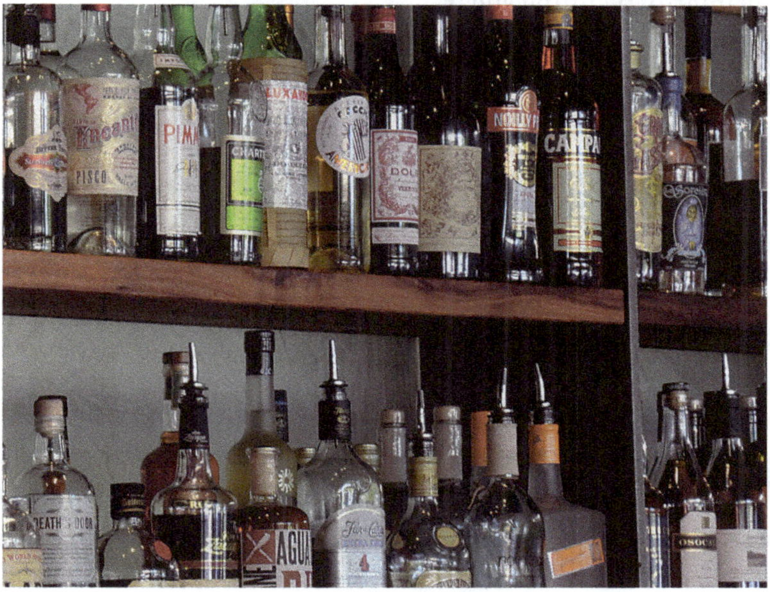

We are not to be trusted. We will lie to you. We will tell you that your outfit matches if we think you are too fragile to hear otherwise. We will tell you how much we enjoyed dinner with your new boyfriend. If we are performing a card trick, we will look you square in the eye and tell you that your card is "lost in the deck," even though we know exactly where to find it.

We will not, however, lie to you when it matters. You will never hear us say, "You're guaranteed to double your money" or "To us, that lump looks harmless." Nor will we try to convince you that cocktails are just as enjoyable under the No Mixer rule. The sad truth is that most cocktails are now off limits.

We have visited nearly all of the famous cocktail lounges in San Francisco. We have stood in line for an hour for a single drink.

We have memorized a password in order to be admitted into a back room "speakeasy." In Argentina, we visited a bar that had to be entered through a florist's walk-in refrigerator. All of this research has reinforced our belief that modern cocktail culture is primarily peddling sugar.

This is not a new problem. We own reproductions of cocktail books dating back to 1882. Nearly every drink listed is sweet enough to be used in a hummingbird feeder.

> **Fact:** The No Mixer rule requires avoiding all added sugar, sweet wines, sweet liquors, pre-made mixers, artificial sweeteners and any more than a small splash of fresh-squeezed juice.

As a result, we estimate that no more than five percent of recognized cocktails are acceptable on the Drink Your Carbs plan.

If you want to enjoy cocktails, you will, by necessity, have to forge a new trail. Experimentation is not without risk, but there are rewards. Some of the drinks you invent will rival the old classics. You will pour some of your creations down the sink. It will not be easy. It will not be cheap. On the bright side, you will still enjoy cocktails without trashing your diet.

To get you started, we created the Drink Your Carbs Cocktail Slot Machine.

Choose one item from each group. Add ice (optional) and take a sip. You will occasionally hit a jackpot. More often then not, you will be left with an empty feeling inside and 25 cents poorer. Just like in a real casino.

> **Fact:** You can't win if you don't play.

The Drink Your Carbs Cocktail Slot Machine

Group 1: Liquor—about 1–1.5 oz.

- Vodka
- Tequila
- Gin
- Whisky
- Scotch
- Grappa
- Sake
- Calvados
- Brandy
- Amaro
- Armagnac
- Other unsweetened alcohols

Group 2: Squeeze/Splash/Muddle

- Lime
- Lemon
- Orange
- Raspberries
- Blueberries
- Mint
- Rosemary
- Lavender
- Bitters
- Pomegranate seeds
- Other fresh fruit
- Basil

Group 3: Finish with—2–3 oz.

- Soda water
- Unsweetened seltzer
- Coffee
- Unsweetened tea

A few examples of successful pulls on the one-armed cocktail bandit:

Whisky
Orange juice
Soda water
Ice

Gin
Lavender (muddled)
Lemon juice
Soda water
Ice
Strain (serve up)

Vodka
Lime juice
Unsweetened tea
Ice

Calvados
(We skipped group two for this cocktail)
Coffee
No ice

A Love Letter to Perfect Cocktail Ice

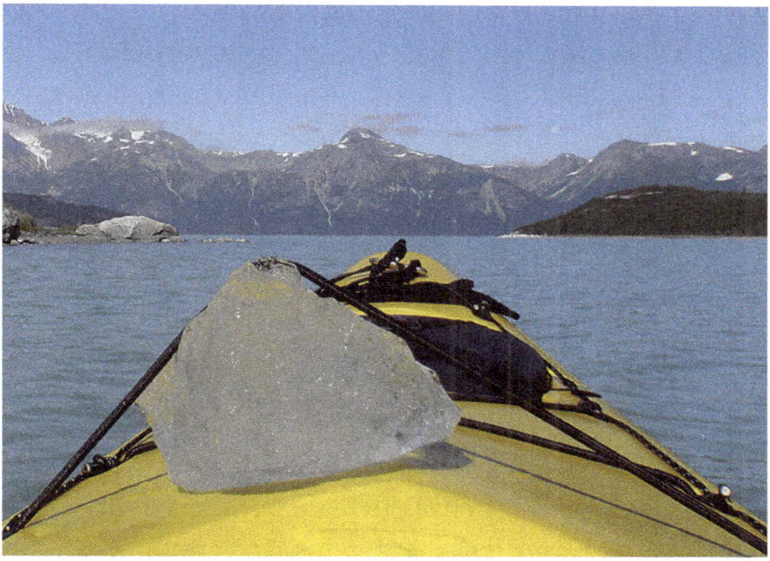

Fact: As you have undoubtedly figured out, you will be drinking most of your hard alcohol straight up, neat, unadulterated or possibly on ice. If you choose to add ice, seek out the best ice you can find, perfectly clear and absolutely flavorless.

We use to laugh at hip bars that insisted on hand-chipping ice from huge blocks, as though ice technology has not advance since the 1800s. No longer. These days, we choose bars solely on the quality of the ice they serve.

Anthony Arendt is a glaciologist in the Geophysical Institute at the University of Alaska. His work is part of a new wave of glacial research. By combining cutting-edge technologies, including satellite gravimetry and airborne laser altimetry with old-fashioned drilling for ice core samples, Arendt is changing our understanding of how glaciers work, why they matter and how they are affected by our warming climate.

Arendt's research often puts him at great personal risk. He was recently stranded on a glacier when his helicopter crashed during a winter storm. Last year, one of Arendt's colleagues fell 75 feet into a crevasse while snowmobiling across a remote glacier. Forget all of the stereotypes of scientists isolated in underground laboratories. Picture instead the X Games with older athletes, less safety equipment and more math.

We didn't contact Dr. Arendt to discuss climate change or any of his important work. We asked him about cocktail ice.

Last year, we travelled to Alaska. We hiked and kayaked around a remote lodge near the city of Homer. We visited friends in Fairbanks (one of whom is the aforementioned glaciologist). We then hopped a small cruise ship into and around Glacier Bay where we discovered that we have, for our entire lives, underestimated the importance of ice.

> **Fact:** Some things go unnoticed until they go terribly wrong. Sewers are an obvious example. We are blind to them right up to the moment that we flush a toilet and, rather than vanishing its contents into the unknown, it begins to overfill. Suddenly, modern sanitation stops being taken for granted and its actual importance comes into sharp relief.
>
> Ice in a cocktail is the opposite. As long as it meets the minimum standard of not tasting fishy, ice goes entirely unnoticed. Would people tolerate a maraschino cherry as cloudy and misshapen as most commercial ice cubes? We think not. We endure mediocre ice

because it barely registers. Ice only stands out when it is truly remarkable.

Alaska's Inside Passage, like many areas where glaciers meet the sea, is littered with small icebergs. Sailing up to Daws Glacier was a little like navigating the waters inside a highball glass. At times, our boat had to push blocks of ice out of the way in order to keep moving. We now have a good idea of what it sounded like when the Titanic hit the iceberg.

Listening to all of that ice clatter against the ship's hull gave Andrea an idea:

Andrea: We should collect an iceberg for happy hour cocktails.

Steven: Is glacier water safe to drink? It could contain viruses from the Ice Age.

Andrea: Have you ever heard of anyone dying from glacier poisoning?

Steven: I don't want to be patient zero in some new plague.

Andrea: Just repeat after me: "I love this plan. I'm excited to be part of it."

Glacier ice is perfectly clear and shatters into jagged shards when struck with a blunt object. It is absolutely flavorless. It is by far the purest ice either of us has ever seen or tasted.

"I'm not an ice physics expert." Dr. Arendt began with this disclaimer when we asked him for the science behind our ice. "I can tell you some general facts that might help."

He then estimated that the ice we collected was at least 100 years old. It began as snow that was then buried in subsequent winters. The pressure from accumulating snow eventually turned our snow into a type of ice glaciologists call "firn." Firn is a Swiss-German term for snow that has been compressed, removing most of the airspace between the individual snowflakes.

"As that ice gets buried deeper and deeper," Dr. Arendt explained, "the pressure goes up and forces those air bubbles out, effectively creating larger ice crystals." It is these large crystals that are the hallmark of glacial ice.

Floating in a drink, the history, science and aesthetics come together to form something greater than all three. The only word we can find to describe the experience is perfect. Until we discovered the crystal clear ice formed under high pressure in the heart of a glacier, we never fully understood the potential for ice to define a cocktail. As far as we are concerned now, the ice is as important as what you chose to pour over it.

> **Fact:** After we returned home, we learned two things; first that we're not the only ones espousing the virtues of the perfection of glacial ice and second, that consuming glacial ice is not entirely without risk. Last year, a man in Patagonia was arrested for stealing 11,453 pounds of ice from Chile's Jorge Montt Glacier. His plan was to sell the ice to upscale bars and restaurants in the capital city, Santiago. He currently awaits trial on charges that include stealing Chile's cultural heritage.[1]

In our defense, no one, including the onboard park ranger, accused us of doing anything untoward. That said, we are still considering printing up bumper stickers that read, "Drinking America's Cultural Heritage Since 2013."

Blooper Reel

Not enough books contain blooper reels. Nearly every Hollywood film now includes, with the credits, footage of the actors and actresses stammering, stuttering and bumping their heads into a boom mic. We don't fully understand the allure, but clearly audiences can't get enough of Robert De Niro giggling uncontrollably. Or, in the case of Jackie Chan, mistiming a stunt and ending up pinned beneath the tires of an 18-wheeler.

This trend has never caught on in literature. Every author acknowledges discarding paragraphs, pages and even whole characters during the editing process. Yet no author we can name has taken the step of including his or her outtakes in a final chapter or appendix.

Imagine how much better *Catcher In The Rye* would have been if we were allowed a glimpse at Salinger's early attempts to write the novel in iambic pentameter.

Who wouldn't enjoy learning that first draft of *Lotita* revolved around the relationship between a young man and an elderly woman à la *Harold and Maude*?

There is no question that reading is in decline. Perhaps more people would be willing to pick up a book if they knew that in the end they would get to see the author walk, metaphorically, into a plate glass window.

Outtakes from Our Research & Writing . . .

Eggs are not dairy products. They are baby chickens. If baby animals are dairy, veal should also be classified as diary.

We have always fancied ourselves as people who could survive a zombie apocalypse. We would hole up underground with the rest of the survivors. During the day we would scavenge food and supplies from the remnants of civilization. At night we would fight off the undead in shifts. It's not a romantic future, but we would do our part to help humanity survive.

Waiting for 20 minutes for a train in the 42nd Street Subway station during rush hour on a blazing summer afternoon has forced us to rethink the plan. The platform was a crush of humanity. What little air there was to breathe was stagnant and foul. If someone had fainted, there was no room to fall.

If surviving a zombie apocalypse demands enduring conditions like those we experienced beneath Times Square, we choose life on the surface.

Even if the undead turn out to be the fast and agile variety rather than the old-school lumbering type, we are still confident that we can out-compete most of them when it comes to hunting brains.

Business Idea: Make tofu hotdogs more authentic by adding rat hairs and insect feces. (It's a little known industry fact that taste and texture are determined by the inclusions.)

Once we have the market cornered, we can sell the sprinkles under the Tofeces® brand name.

The first edition of The Paleo Diet by Dr. Loren Cordain proudly declares that his diet protects against "Syndrome X."[1] Today, the term "Metabolic Syndrome" is used to describe the standard package of obesity-related illnesses, ranging from high blood pressure to Type-2 Diabetes. When Cordain published his diet in 2002, the term was not yet in popular use. Cordain instead referred to that group of symptoms and diseases as "Syndrome X."

We love "Syndrome X" because it sounds like something out of a comic book. We know what Cordain intended, nonetheless, we cannot read the words "Syndrome X" without picturing a meeting of the Super Friends.

Superman: This meeting has been called to order. Will someone second the motion?

Aquaman: I second the motion to officially open this meeting of the Super Friends.

Superman: All in favor? Great. We do have one change to the agenda. Batman was planning to walk us through how to use the secret decoder ring, but we'll have to table it until next week. Right now we need to deal with Syndrome X, which is threating to turn the human population of this planet into turtles.

Wonder Woman: I wish you'd stop talking like that.

Superman: Like what?

Wonder Woman: Like you're somehow separate from the rest of the population.

Superman: What the hell are you talking about!? I am separate from the rest of the population.

Robin: I'd like to make a motion that we table Syndrome X until we're able to discuss it using our inside voices. Flash, can you second that so we can move on to the decoder ring?

Colonel Oliver North taught us that you can't be indicted if you've shredded all the evidence. You occasionally lose track of something you wish you had, but the tradeoff is worth it. Had Richard Nixon been a shredder instead of a hoarder, he would've been able to gracefully retire from the Presidency into a life of organized crime, just like Dick Cheney.

There are signs that the obesity epidemic is slowing. But the statisticians making this argument discount future innovations of the Snack Food Industrial Complex. In other words, in an underground laboratory somewhere in the Midwest, scientists are very likely developing a Snickers bar in an irresistible shade of blue.

We are not conspiracy buffs, but if Drink Your Carbs really catches on we expect to be assassinated by the Frito-Lay Corporation.

Spicing up you sex life with whipped cream negates all exercise benefits. A half hour in the sack burns around 85 calories which is, coincidentally, the exact same number of calories as in half a cup of pressurized whipped cream.

The Michelin Man made his first appearance in a French advertising poster in 1894. The original Michelin Man smoked cigars, wore pince-nez glasses and was made up of narrow segments designed to be reminiscent of bicycle tires. To our eyes he looks like a pompous, overweight Egyptian mummy. The Michelin Man also had a name: "Bibendum." That name is still used, but only by advertising executives and designers of crossword puzzles.

Bibendum has since undergone numerous, Michael Jackson-like transformations. In the early 1900s, he briefly turned black. Somewhere along the line, he quit smoking and had his eyes fixed. In 1998, the Michelin Corporation slimmed him down and gave him more definition in his chest and shoulders. Speculation at the time pinned the fitness overhaul on the fact that in Spain, the word "Michelin" was used as slang for "belly fat" or "spare tire."

Normally we don't go quite this far afield in our adjunct facts. But we think it's fascinating that, as industrialized countries have grown more obese, the Michelin Man has become visibly slimmer. If current trends continue, Bibendum will sprout six-pack abs on the exact same day the last person on earth develops Type-2 Diabetes.

The Best Medical Advice We Have Ever Received: Over 10 years ago, we were in line at a wine tasting in Paso Robles, California. Dr. Seymour Alban happened to be standing in front of us. Dr. Alban was in his seventies at the time. He was still practicing medicine. Dr. Alban's advice came in the form of an answer to a question we no longer remember. "I'm a doctor," he said, "and I'm telling you to drink more wine."

Acknowledgments

Drink Your Carbs was written like Amish communities raise a barn. It would not have been possible without the help and support of nearly everyone we know.

Here are a few of the many who aided and abetted us along the way.

Our editor, Dan Seligson. We understand that it is not customary to laugh out loud while reading an editor's comments. Tears and flashes of rage are, apparently, the norm. Dan edited no fewer than three drafts of this book. He contributed countless jokes along with all of his other comments and insights. This book is far better for Dan having been a part of it.

Our design team is unequaled. Without this talented group, Drink Your Carbs would be a hand-stapled, photocopied zine. We offer special thanks to:

Nicole Delmage;
Misa Erder;
Kate Havran;
Jennifer Omner;
Boyd Richard;
Alana Shaw.

Our friends and family deserve huge thanks for their ideas, jokes, facts, recipes and exercise routines. They freely shared their personal stories and allowed us to use their real names. Sometimes we questioned their sanity, but we never questioned their love. This includes (but, as they say in the legal world, is not limited to):

Anthony Arendt and Kristen Barton;
David Bayendor;
Dirk Bird;
Stephanie Boyden;
Jennifer Collins;
The Deutsch family;
Gary Donner and Irene Miller;
Elliott Downing;
Dave Elger;
Andrea Frizzi and Tara Meekma-Frizzi;
Patrick Green;
Willie and Connie Hector;
David E. Hedges II;
Gen Izutsu;
Kari Kelly;
Christopher Lawson;
Paul Lewis;
Bentley Lim;
Amulya Malladi;
David Marlow;
Christopher McCown and Rebecca Stanfield McCown;
Andrea Plastas and Joyce Lupac;
Cassandra Seebaum and Shawn Hector;
Lyle Seebaum;
The Seebaum, Haldeman, Shaw, Fox and Hector families;
Josh and Pierrete Silverman;
Susan Hunt Stevens;
Jessamin Swearingen;
Jon Taylor and Peter Waterloo;
Tricia, Emma, Annie and John Tilley;

Monica Ward and Natascha Seideneck;

Jenny Werba, Trent Simmons and The United Barbell Community;

Mike Wolfson;

Scott Yonehiro.

Last, but certainly not least, we give our tremendous gratitude to all our other friends and supporters who are too numerous to name. You caught our typos. You corrected our facts. You shared our Tweets and Facebook posts, effectively spamming your entire community on our behalf. You defended us when we were accused of being morons and/or promoting *drunkorexia*. You never shied away from the difficult task of telling us that something sucked. And most of all, you encouraged us to keep writing.

To all of you: a mixer-free cheers!

Drink Your Carbs was made possible, in part, by a generous grant from Feldman's Kosher Seafood.

Notes

Listed below are the key journal articles, books, websites and other materials we used in creating Drink Your Carbs.

All of the websites cited match the content we describe as of March 28, 2014. Unfortunately, this provides no guarantee that the content will not have been replaced by cat videos by the time you get there. If you need one of our online sources—for example, your PhD dissertation stands or falls based on one of our "facts"—drop us a line. We very likely have a screenshot.

Introduction: What Is Drink Your Carbs?

1. Penn State University. "Americans Fall Short of Federal Exercise Recommendations." *Penn State News*, May 8, 2012. http://news.psu.edu/story/149052/2012/05/08/americans-fall-short-federal-exercise-recommendations.
2. Johnson, Rachel K. et al. "Dietary Sugars Intake and Cardiovascular Health: A Scientific Statement from the American Heart Association." *Journal of the American Heart Association* 120 (2009): 1011.

One: How Diets Work

1. Atkins, Robert C. *Dr. Atkins' New Diet Revolution* (New York: Avon, 1992), 9.
2. Ornish, Dr. Dean. "Atkins Diet Increases All-Cause Mortality." *Huffington Post*, September 7, 2010. http://www.huffingtonpost.com/dr-dean-ornish/an-atkins-diet-increases-_b_707005.html.

3. Pritikin, Nathan. *The Pritikin Permanent Weight-Loss Manual* (New York: Bantam, 1981), 7–11.
4. Agatson, Authur. *The South Beach Diet* (New York: Rodale, 2003), 9.
5. Parker, Hillary. "A Sweet Problem: Princeton Researchers Find that High-Fructose Corn Syrup Prompts Considerably More Weight Gain." *News at Princeton*, March 12, 2010. http://www.princeton.edu/main/news/archive/S26/91/22K07/index.xml?section=topstories.
6. Park, Madison. "Twinkie Diet Helps Nutrition Professor Lose 27 Pounds." *CNN Health*, November 8, 2010. http://www.cnn.com/2010/HEALTH/11/08/twinkie.diet.professor/.
7. Ebbeling, Cara B. et al. "Effects of Dietary Composition on Energy Expenditure During Weight-Loss Maintenance." *Journal of the American Medical Association* 307 (2012): 2627–2634.
8. Foster, Gary D. et al. "Weight and Metabolic Outcomes After 2 Years on a Low-Carbohydrate Versus Low-Fat Diet: A Randomized Trial." *Annals of Internal Medicine* 153 (2010): 147–157.
9. Atkins, Robert C. *Dr. Atkins' New Diet Revolution* (New York: Avon, 1992), 58.
10. Boston Medical Center. "Nutrition and Weight Management." http://www.bmc.org/nutritionweight/services/weightmanagement.htm.

Two: Why Are Americans Fat?

1. Begley, Sharon. "Fat and Getting Fatter: U.S. Obesity Rates to Soar by 2030." *Reuters*, September 18, 2012. http://www.reuters.com/article/2012/09/18/us-obesity-us-idUSBRE88H0RA20120918.

2. Washington Post. "The History of the Food Pyramid." Last modified January 31, 2011. http://www.washingtonpost.com/wp-srv/special/health/food-pyramid/.

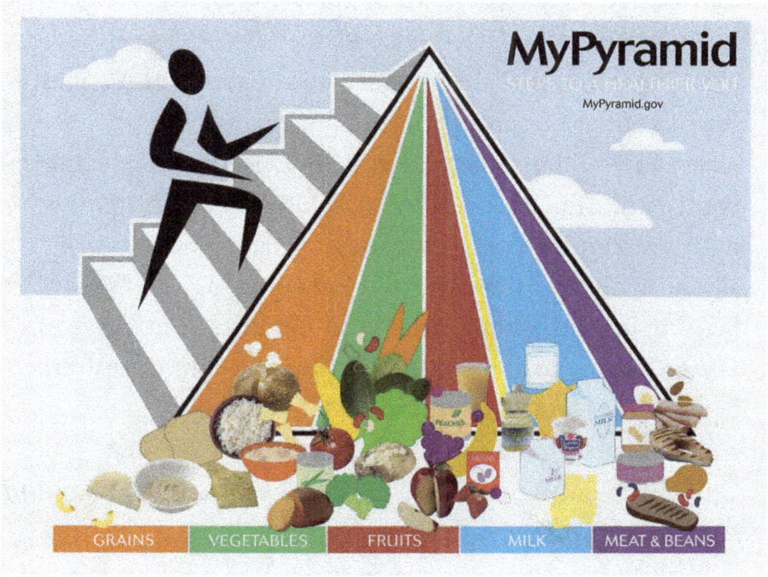

My ~~Little Pony~~ Pyramid, 2005

3. United States Department of Agriculture. "MyPlate and Historical Food Pyramid Resources." *Center for Nutrition Policy and Promotion* (1996): 4–5.
4. The Washington Post. "The History of the Food Pyramid."
5. The theory that the world is run by Reptile People can be found in the work of author and crazy person David Icke. Icke alleges that the President, members of the British Royal Family and pretty much everyone else who holds power or money is actually a disguised reptile from the Constellation Draco. Normally we would offer a citation, but in this case

we can't do that. The last thing we want to do is to help sell even a single copy of one of his angry, paranoid books.

Also, please don't listen to Icke when he accuses us of being part of the hidden reptile conspiracy. We assure you that we are 100 percent human, even though, as Icke is certain to point out, that is exactly what a reptile would say.

6. U.S. Department of Commerce. "1992 Census of Agriculture." *Bureau of the Census* (1992): 1–2.
7. Neuman, William. "Nutrition Plate Unveiled, Replacing Food Pyramid." *New York Times*, June 2, 2011. http://www.nytimes.com/2011/06/03/business/03plate.html?_r=0.
8. Khan, Amina. "Farewell, Food Pyramid—USDA is Now Serving up Nutritional Advice on My Plate." *Los Angeles Times*, June 2, 2011. http://articles.latimes.com/2011/jun/02/news/la-heb-food-pyramid-my-plate-20110602.
9. United States Department of Agriculture. "Dietary Guidelines For Americans." *Center For Nutrtion Policy and Promotion* (2011): 8.

   (This language was removed from the SuperTracker website, but it can still be found in the reference above.)

Four: Three Simple Steps to Get Started Now

1. Nielsen, Samara Joy et al. "Calories Consumed from Alcoholic Beverages by U.S. Adults, 2007–2010." *Centers for Disease Control and Prevention National Center for Health Statistics* 110 (2012): 1–8.
2. Radcliffe, Shawn. "The Cost of Drinking: 10 Extra Pounds of Fat a Year?" *Men's Fitness*. http://www.mensfitness.com/nutrition/what-to-drink/effects-of-drinking-extra-pounds.
3. Gastaldelli, Amalia. "Abdominal Fat: Does it Predict the Development of Type 2 Diabetes?" *American Journal of Clinical Nutrition* 87 (2008): 1118–1119.

Six: The Basic Drink Your Carbs Food List

1. U.S. Food and Drug Administration. "What You Need to Know About Mercury in Fish and Shellfish." Last modified June 24, 2013. http://www.fda.gov/food/resourcesforyou/consumers/ucm110591.htm.
2. Monterey Bay Aquarium Seafood Watch. "Seafood Recommendations." http://www.seafoodwatch.org/cr/cr_seafoodwatch/sfw_recommendations.aspx.
3. Ross, Robert Alan. "The Science of Raw Food." http://www.rawfoodlife.com/.

Thirteen: What about Gluten and Dairy?

1. Braly, James and Ron Hoggan. *Dangerous Grains: Why Gluten Cereal Grains May be Hazardous to Your Health* (New York: Avery Trade, 2002), Kindle edition free sample.
2. Wolf, Robb. *The Paleo Solution: The Original Human Diet* (Las Vegas: Victory Belt Publishing, 2010), 94–95.
3. Freedman, Rory and Kim Barnouin. *Skinny Bitch* (Philidephia: Running Press, 2005), Kindle edition.
4. National Dairy Council. "Nutrition Education Resources." Last modified 2005. http://school.fueluptoplay60.com/tools/nutrition-education/view.php?id=23445811.

Fifteen: How Much Can I Drink?

1. United States Department of Agriculture. "Dietary Guidelines For Americans, 2010." *Center For Nutrtion Policy and Promotion* (2011): 21.
2. International Center For Alcohol Policies. "International Drinking Guidelines." Last modified February 2010. http://www.icap.org/table/Internationaldrinkingguidelines.

The International Center For Alcohol Policies lists all alcohol consumption numbers in grams of pure alcohol.

While this makes it easy to compare different countries' recommendations, this can make it difficult to figure out how much you are personally consuming. The best resource we have found for converting grams of alcohol into recognizable drinks is Wikipedia: http://en.wikipedia.org/wiki/Standard_drink.

3. World Health Organization. "Global Status Report on Alcohol and Health 2011." Last modified February 11, 2011. http://www.who.int/substance_abuse/publications/global_alcohol_report/en/index.html.
4. National Institutes of Health. "Moderate and Binge Drinking." http://www.niaaa.nih.gov/alcohol-health/overview-alcohol-consumption/moderate-binge-drinking.
5. Adams, Stephen. "Alcohol Guidelines 'Too High' Say Doctors." *Telegraph*, January 1, 2013. http://www.telegraph.co.uk/health/healthnews/9774223/Alcohol-guidelines-too-high-say-doctors.html.
6. International Center For Alcohol Policies. "Policy Tools: 'Binge' Drinking." http://www.icap.org/policytools/icapbluebook/bluebookmodules/6bingedrinking/tabid/167/default.aspx.
7. Deutsch, Steven H. "Red, White and Green: A Study in the Successful Importation of Popular Culture from the Non-English Speaking World into the American Cultural Identity." Master's thesis, University of Denver, 1998.

Sixteen: Artificial and Alternative Sweeteners

1. United States Environmental Protection Agency. "EPA Removes Saccharin from Hazardous Substances Listing." Last modified December 14, 2010. http://yosemite.epa.gov/opa/admpress.nsf/d0cf6618525a9efb85257359003fb69d/ea895a11ea50a56d852577f9005e2690!OpenDocument.
2. Dunn, Rob. "Human Ancestors Were Nearly All

Vegetarians." *Scientific American*, July 23, 2012. http://blogs.scientificamerican.com/guest-blog/2012/07/23/human-ancestors-were-nearly-all-vegetarians.

Nineteen: Exercise: A Necessary Evil

1. Ornish, Dean. *Dr. Dean Ornish's Program for Reversing Heart Disease* (New York: Ivy, 1996), 316.
2. Atkins, Robert C. *Dr. Atkins' New Diet Revolution* (New York: Avon, 1992), 256–264.
3. United States Department of Agriculture. "What is Physical Activity?" http://www.choosemyplate.gov/physical-activity/what.html.

Twenty: Basic Exercise

1. Hall, Cameron et al. "Energy Expenditure of Walking and Running: Comparison with Prediction Equations." *Medicine & Science in Sports & Exercise* 36 (2004): 2128–2134.
2. Ibid.
3. McMillen, Matt. "Interval Training Burns More Calories in Less Time." *WebMD,* October 12, 2012. http://www.webmd.com/fitness-exercise/news/20121012/interval-training-burns-more-calories-less-time.
4. Jones, Laura S. "Cardio versus Weights: The Battle Is Over." *Washington Post*, April 24, 2007. http://www.washingtonpost.com/wp-dyn/content/article/2007/04/20/AR2007042001772.html.

Twenty One: Advanced Exercise

1. Fell, James S. "The Myth of Ripped Muscles and Calorie Burns." *Los Angeles Times*, May 16, 2011. http://articles.latimes.com/2011/may/16/health/la-he-fitness-muscle-myth-20110516.
2. Fleck, SJ and Falkel, JE. "Value of Resistance Training For

The Reduction Of Sports Injuries." *Sports Medicine* 3 (1986): 61–8.

3. Hamill, Brian P. "Relative Safety of Weightlifting and Weight Training." *Journal of Strength and Conditioning Research* 8 (1994): 53–57.
4. If this example sounds oddly specific, that's because it is. Our editor, Dan, did this to himself a few years back. We know about it because he penciled his tale of woe into the margin of an early draft of this book.
5. American Physiological Society. "Minutes of Hard Exercise Can Lead to All-Day Calorie Burn." Last modified October 10, 2012. http://www.the-aps.org/mm/hp/Audiences/Public-Press/For-the-Press/releases/12/37.html.
6. Ritsumeikan University. "Interview with the Founder of the World-Renowned Tabata Protocol." http://www.ritsumei.ac.jp/eng/html/research/areas/feat-researchers/interview/izumi_t.html.

Twenty Two: Insane Exercise

1. Nelson, Toben F. and Henry Wechsler. "Alcohol and college athletes." *Medicine & Science In Sports & Exercise* 33 (2001): 43–47.
2. O'Brien, Kerry S., Joshua M. Blackie and John A. Hunter. "Hazardous Drinking in Elite New Zealand Sportspeople." *Alcohol & Alcoholism* 40 (2005): 239–241.
3. Barnes, Matthew J., Toby Mündel and Stephen R. Stannard. "Acute Alcohol Consumption Aggravates the Decline in Muscle Performance Following Strenuous Eccentric Exercise." *Journal of Science and Medicine in Sport* 13 (2010): 189–193.
4. Ibid.
5. Brown University. "Alcohol and Your Body." http://brown.edu/Student_Services/Health_Services/Health_Education/

alcohol,_tobacco,_&_other_drugs/alcohol/alcohol_&_your_body.php.
6. Barnes et al. "Acute. . ."
7. Ibid.
8. Barnes, Matthew J., Toby Mundel and Stephen R. Stannard. "A Low Dose of Alcohol Does Not Impact Skeletal Muscle Performance After Exercise-Induced Muscle Damage." *European Journal of Applied Physiology* 111 (2011): 725–729.
9. Clarkson, Pricilla M. and Freida Reichsman. "The Effect of Ethanol on Exercise-Induced Muscle Damage." *Journal of Studies on Alcohol* 51 (1990): 19–23.
10. Ibid.
11. Castillo, Manuel J. "BEER AFTER EXERCISE: Yes or No?" Paper presented at the European Conference on Nutrition, Madrid, Spain, October 28, 2011.
12. Centers for Disease Control and Prevention. "Alcohol and Public Health: Frequently Asked Questions." Last modified March 14, 2014. http://www.cdc.gov/alcohol/faqs.htm#drinkDrive.

Twenty Six: Travel to New York, New York

1. Flynn, Dan. "Still Too Many Raw Oyster Deaths in Gulf States" *Food Safety News*, November 22, 2011. http://www.foodsafetynews.com/2011/11/still-too-many-raw-oyster-deaths/#.Uin_-hY2W6E.
2. Cordain, Loren Ph.D. *The Paleo Diet: Lose Weight and Get Healthy by Eating the Foods You Were Designed to Eat* (New York: John Wiley & Sons, 2002), 110–112.

Twenty Seven: Travel to Antarctica

1. Wikipedia. "Antarctica." http://en.wikipedia.org/wiki/Antarctica.
2. Department of the Environment Australian Antarctic

Division. "How Many People Live in Antarctica?" Last modified March 11, 2003. http://www.antarctica.gov.au/about-antarctica/people-in-antarctica/how-many.

Twenty Nine: Travel to Crete, Greece

1. Faculty of the Harvard School of Public Health. "Center for Global Tobacco Control." *Harvard School of Public Health* (2011): 17–20
2. Vardavas, Constantine I. and Anthony G. Kafatos. "Smoking Policy and Prevalence in Greece: An Overview." *European Journal of Public Health* 17 (2006): 211–213.

Thirty: Case Study

1. Vandewater, Elizabeth A, Mi-suk Shim and Allison G Caplovitz. "Linking Obesity and Activity Level with Children's Television and Video Game Use." *Journal of Adolescence* 27 (2004): 71–85.

Thirty One: A History Of Drinker's Diets

1. Banting, William. *Letter on Corpulence, Addressed to the Public* (London: Harrison, 1864), 1–50.
2. Gardener, Jameson and Elliot Williams. *The Drinking Man's Diet* (San Francisco: Cameron & Co., 1964), 1–50.
3. Time Magazine Editorial Staff. "Dieting: The Drinking Man's Danger." *Time Magazine*, March 5, 1965. http://content.time.com/time/magazine/article/0,9171,839328,00.html.
4. Carl, Lüc. *The Drunk Diet: How I Lost 40 Pounds . . . Wasted* (New York: St. Martin's Press, 2012), Kindle edition.

Thirty Two: Recipes

1. Wolf, Robb. *The Paleo Solution: The Original Human Diet* (Las Vegas: Victory Belt, 2010), 98.
2. Ibid., 240.

Recipes: The Burger Salad

1. United States Department of Agriculture. "Cooking Meat? Check the New Recommended Temperatures." Last modified May 25, 2011. http://blogs.usda.gov/2011/05/25/cooking-meat-check-the-new-recommended-temperatures/.
2. Food Network. "Meat and Poultry Temperature Guide." http://www.foodnetwork.com/recipes-and-cooking/meat-and-poultry-temperature-guide/index.html.
3. Lagasse, Emeril. "Steak Tartare." *Food Network*. http://www.foodnetwork.com/recipes/emeril-live/steak-tartare-recipe/index.html.

Recipes: Chicken alla Milanese

1. Taipei Times. "Keeping a Secret Secret for the Colonel." Last modified July 31, 2005. http://web.archive.org/web/20060113220400/http://www.taipeitimes.com/News/bizfocus/archives/2005/07/31/2003265834.

Recipes: Drink Your Carbs Brownies

1. Amsterdam, Elana. "Brownies." Last modified February 24, 2009. http://www.elanaspantry.com/brownies.
2. Courson, Kelly. "Peanut Butter Love." Last modified January 30, 2007. http://www.celiacchicks.com/gluten-free-recipes/peanut_butter_l.html.

Thirty Three: Cocktails

Cocktails: A Love Letter to Perfect Cocktail Ice

1. The Week. "The Man Who Stole a Glacier . . . To Make Cocktails?" Last modified February 6, 2012. http://theweek.com/article/index/224082/the-man-who-stole-a-glaciernbsp-to-make-cocktails.

Blooper Reel

1. Cordain, Loren Ph.D. *The Paleo Diet: Lose Weight and Get Healthy by Eating the Foods You Were Designed to Eat* (New York: John Wiley & Sons, 2002), 75.

About the Authors

Steven Deutsch and Andrea Seebaum

We have known each other since middle school. We were friends through high school and college. A few years after graduating, we looked at one another and thought, "When did you get cute?" We never looked back. In 2014, we celebrated our 17th wedding anniversary.

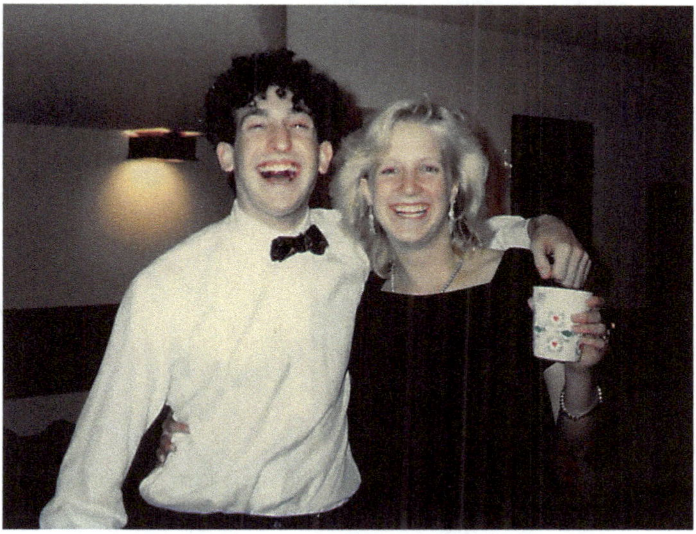

Steven and Andrea, 1989

These days, we reside in Northern California where we drink, cook, CrossFit, eat out way too often and make small quantities of wine under the ThoseFuckers label.

www.ingramcontent.com/pod-product-compliance
Lightning Source LLC
Chambersburg PA
CBHW060025030426
42334CB00019B/2180
* 9 7 8 0 9 9 0 4 4 9 6 1 4 *